Fibrin Sealing in Surgical and Nonsurgical Fields

Volume 2

G. Schlag H.-W. Waclawiczek
R. Daum (Eds.)

General and Abdominal Surgery Pediatric Surgery

With 110 Figures and 41 Tables

Springer-Verlag
Berlin Heidelberg New York
London Paris Tokyo
Hong Kong Barcelona
Budapest

Prof. Dr. GÜNTHER SCHLAG

Ludwig-Boltzmann-Institute
for Experimental and Clinical Traumatology
Donaueschingenstraße 13, 1200 Wien
Austria

Prof. Dr. H.-W. WACLAWICZEK

Landeskrankenanstalten Salzburg
Ist Surgery Department
Müllner Hauptstraße 48, 5020 Salzburg
Austria

Prof. Dr. R. DAUM

Ruprecht-Karls-University Heidelberg
Clinic of Surgery
Dept. for Pediatric Surgery
Im Neuenheimer Feld 110, 69120 Heidelberg
Germany

ISBN-13: 978-3-540-57742-3 **e-ISBN-13: 978-3-642-85101-8**
DOI: 10.1007/978-3-642-85101-8

CIP data applied for

Softcover reprint of the hardcover 1st edition 1994

Typesetting: Mitterweger, 68723 Plankstadt
Printing and Binding: Zechnersche Buchdruckerei, 67346 Speyer
23/3145 5 4 3 2 1 0 – Printed on acid-free paper.

Preface

These eight volumes, which developed out of the international congress "Update and Future Trends in Fibrin Sealing in Surgical and Nonsurgical Fields" held in November 1992, present the state of the art in fibrin sealing. Initially, fibrin sealant played an important role in surgery. During the past few years, it has been increasingly applied in nonsurgical applications and we can now say that it has become an integral component of medical treatment.

The doubts which have been raised by nonusers about the efficacy of fibrin sealant are no longer valid. The correct indication and technique continue to be basic prerequisites for effective treatment. Even today – 20 years after fibrin sealant was first used – the three most prominent effects of fibrin sealant are still hemostasis, sealing of the wound, and support of wound healing.

The problems posed by the transmission of viral infections have gained substantially in importance because of the potential transmission of AIDS via fibrin sealant. Fortunately, this is so unlikely today that it no longer represents a cause for concern, which does not mean, however, that research in this field can be discontinued.

Seven years have passed since the last series of books on fibrin sealing were published. Since then many new results have been obtained, in particular in the field of gastrointestinal surgery. From the beginnings of fibrin sealing, general and abdominal surgery have been among its main indications. Since then the application of fibrin sealant in routine intestinal anastomoses has become less important than its application in high risk anastomoses (colorectal, jejuno-esophageal). During the past years fibrin sealant has also often been used to secure vascular anastomoses, in particular after liver transplantation. Another important indication for fibrin sealant in abdominal surgery is the treatment of fistulas and lymphatic fistulas.

In pediatric surgery fibrin sealant is increasingly being applied in new areas, among these, a special indication is orthotopic liver transplantation. The frequent use of fibrin sealant to improve surgery of parenchymatous organs (liver, spleen, pancreas, and kidney) has led to further perfection of the technique and to other important applications. We, the editors, would like to thank all the authors for their cooperation and excellent contributions and photographs. Their work has made publication of these eight volumes on fibrin sealing possible. Special thanks are due to Dr. V. Gebhardt and his expert colleagues for efficient and constructive cooperation in the publication of these books at the Springer publishing company and to Gudrun Schrodt for her untiring efforts in obtaining manuscripts, proof reading, and corresponding with the authors.

G. Schlag
H. W. Waclawiczek
R. Daum

Contents

List of Contributors

ALDINI, N. N.
Exp. Surg. Dept. I.O.R., Univ. of Bologna, I-40136 Bologna, Italy

ALFANI, D.
II. Patol. Spec. Chir. Univ. di Roma "La Sapienza",
I-00167 Rome, Italy

BADELLINO, F.
Div. di Oncol. Chir. Instit. Nazion. per la Ricerca sul Cancro,
Viale B.XV, I-16132 Genoa, Italy

BALSELLS, J.
H-P-B and Liver Transplant. Univ. Dept. of Surg. Hospital General
Vall d'Hebron, Univ. Autónoma, E-08035 Barcelona, Spain

BECKER, Ch.
Klinik für Kinder- und Neugeborenen Chirurgie, Westfälische-
Wilhelms-Universität, Albert-Schweitzer-Straße 33,
D-48149 Münster, Federal Republic of Germany

BERLOCO, P.
II. Patol. Spec. Chir. Univ. di Roma "La Sapienza",
I-00167 Rome, Italy

BOECKL, O.
1st Surg. Dept. LKA Salzburg, Müllner Hauptstr. 48,
A-5020 Salzburg, Austria

BOERSCH, G.
Med. Klinik, Elisabeth-Krankenhaus, Akad. Lehrkrankenhaus,
Univ. Essen, GHS
Moltkestraße 61, D-45138 Essen, Federal Republic of Germany

BOIXOCHOA, J.
Ped. Surg. Dept., Hosp. Infantil Valle d'Hebron,
E-08035 Barcelona, Spain

BRANDS, W.
Kinderchirurgische Klinik, Städtisches Klinikum Karlsruhe,
Karl-Wilhelm-Str. 1, D-76131 Karlsruhe, Federal Republic
of Germany

Bruzzone, P.
II. Patol. Spec. Chir. Univ. di Roma “La Sapienza”,
I-00167 Rome, Italy

Caffarena, P. E.
Univ. of Genoa „G. Gaslini” Inst. Genoa, Largo G. Gaslini, 5,
I-16148 Genoa, Italy

Canavese, G.
Div. di Oncol. Chir. Instit. Nazion. per la Ricerca sul Cancro,
Viale B.XV, I-16132 Genoa, Italy

Carboni, F.
II. Patol. Spec. Chir. Univ. di Roma “La Sapienza”,
I-00167 Rome, Italy

Caricato, M.
II. Patol. Spec. Chir. Univ. di Roma “La Sapienza”,
I-00167 Rome, Italy

Cavallini, M.
Dept. of Surg., 1° Instit. di Clin. Chir., Univ. of Rome,
“La Sapienza”, I-00167 Rome, Italy

Catturich, A.
Div. di Oncol. Chir. Instit. Nazion. per la Ricerca sul Cancro,
Viale B.XV, I-16132 Genoa, Italy

Charco, R.
H-P-B and Liver Transplant. Univ. Dept. of Surg. Hospital General
Vall d’Hebron, Univ. Autónoma, E-08035 Barcelona, Spain

Cortesini, R.
II. Patol. Spec. Chir. Univ. di Roma “La Sapienza”,
I-00167 Rome, Italy

Daum, R.
Dept. of Ped. Surg., Univ. of Heidelberg, Im Neuenheimer Feld 110,
D-69120 Heidelberg, Federal Republic of Germany

De Dreuzy, O.
Dept. de Péd., Univ. Paris Sud, CHU de Bicêtre,
78 Rue du Général Leclerc, F-94275 Kremlin Bicêtre, France

Degenhardt, P.
Kinderchir. Abt., St. Elisabethklinik Saarlouis
D-66740 Saarlouis, Federal Republic of Germany

Denno, R.
1st Dept. of Surg. Sapporo Med. Coll., S. I. W. 16, Chuo-ku,
Sapporo, 060 Japan

Diaz, A.
H-P-B and Liver Transplant. Univ. Dept. of Surg. Hospital General
Vall d’Hebron, Univ. Autónoma, E-08035 Barcelona, Spain

Di Somma, C.
Dept. de Péd., Univ. Paris Sud, CHU de Bicêtre,
78 Rue du Général Leclerc, F-94275 Kremlin Bicêtre, France

Edo, A.
H-P-B and Liver Transplant. Univ. Dept. of Surg. Hospital General
Vall d'Hebron, Univ. Autónoma, E-08035 Barcelona, Spain

Fernández Ruiz, M.
San Millán Hospital, Serv. de Chir., Autonomia de la Rioja 3,
E-26004 Logrono, Spain

Fíger, J.
2nd Dept. of Surg. Med. Faculty Comenius Univ., Bezrucova 5,
CSRF-815 26 Bratislava

Fini, M.
Exp. Surg. Dept. I.O.R., Univ. of Bologna, I-40136 Bologna, Italy

Friedl, P. G.
Surgery Department, Universität Heidelberg, Im Neuenheimer
Feld 110, D-69120 Heidelberg, Federal Republic of Germany

Gauthier, F.
Dept. de Péd., Univ. Paris Sud, CHU de Bicêtre,
78 Rue du Général Leclerc, F-94275 Kremlin Bicêtre, France

Gdanietz, K.
Kinderchirurgische Klinik, Klinikum Berlin-Buch,
Karower Straße 11, D-13125 Berlin, Federal Republic of Germany

Giardino, M.
Exp. Surg. Dept. I.O.R., Univ. of Bologna, I-40136 Bologna, Italy

Giavaresi, G.
Exp. Surg. Dept. I.O.R., Univ. of Bologna, I-40136 Bologna, Italy

Gipponi, M.
Div. di Oncol. Chir. Instit. Nazion. per la Ricerca sul Cancro,
Viale B.XV, I-16132 Genoa, Italy

Gutsche, I.
Kinderchirurgische Klinik, Klinikum Berlin-Buch,
Karower Straße 11, D-13125 Berlin, Federal Republic of Germany

Herfarth, Ch.
Surgery Department, Universität Heidelberg, Im Neuenheimer
Feld 110, D-69120 Heidelberg, Federal Republic of Germany

Hebrero San Martin, J.
San Millán Hospital, Serv. de Chir, Autonomia de la Rioja 3,
E-26004 Logrono, Spain

Hirata, K.
1st Dept. of Surg. Sapporo Med. Coll. S. 1, W. 16, Chuo-ku,
Sapporo, 060 Japan

Hirohashi, K.
2nd Dept. of Surg., Osaka City Univ. Med. School, I-5-7,
Asahi-machi, Abono-ku, Osaka 545, Japan

Iacconi, P.
Cattedra di Endocrinochir., Clin. Chir. dell' Univ. di Pisa,
v. Roma 67, CAP 56100 Pisa, Italy

Jahn, S.
Kinderchir. Abt., St. Elisabethklinik Saarlouis,
D-66740 Saarlouis, Federal Republic of Germany

Jasonni, V.
Univ. of Genoa "G. Gaslini" Inst. Genoa, Largo G. Gaslini, 5,
I-16148 Genoa, Italy

Katsuramaki, T.
1st Dept. of Surg. Sapporo Med. Coll., S. 1, W. 16, Chuo-ku,
Sapporo, 060 Japan

Kimura, H.
1st Dept. of Surg. Sapporo Med. Coll., S. 1, W. 16, Chuo-ku,
Sapporo, 060 Japan

Kirchmair, F.
Kinderchir. Abt., St. Elisabethklinik Saarlouis,
D-66740 Saarlouis, Federal Republic of Germany

Kinoshita, H.
2nd Dept. of Surg., Osaka City Univ. Med. School, 1-5-7,
Asahi-machi, Abeno-ku, Osaka 545, Japan

Kroiss, A.
2nd Department of Surgery, Universität Wien, Spitalgasse 23,
A-1090 Wien

Kubo, S.
2nd Dept. of Surg., Osaka City Univ. Med. School, 1-5-7,
Asahi-machi, Abeno-ku, Osaka 545, Japan

Lababidi, A.
Dept. de Péd., Univ. Paris Sud, CHU de Bicêtre,
78 Rue du Général Leclerc, F-94275 Kremlin Bicêtre, France

Labenz, J.
Medizinische Klinik, Elisabeth-Krankenhaus, Akademisches
Lehrkrankenhaus, Universität Essen, Moltkestraße 61,
D-45138 Essen, Federal Republic of Germany

Labuda, M.
2nd Dept. of Surg. Med. Faculty Comenius Univ., Bezrucova 5,
CSRF-815 26 Bratislava

Lázaro, J. L.
II-P-B and Liver Transplant. Univ. Dept. of Surg. Hospital General
Vall d'Hebron, Univ. Autónoma, E-08035 Barcelona, Spain

LELLI CHIESA, P. L.
Dept. of Ped. Surg., Univ. of Genoa "G. Gaslini" Inst. Genoa, Largo G. Gaslini, 5, I-16148 Genoa, Italy

MAIER, W. A.
Fridtjof Nansen Straße 58, D-76228 Karlsruhe, Federal Republic of Germany

MAKAIOVÁ, I.
Clin. of Nuclear Med., Nat. Oncol. Inst. CSRF-815 26 Bratislava

MARCZELL, A. P.
Department of Surgery, Hanusch-Medical-Center, Heinrich-Collin-Straße 30, A-1140 Wien, Austria

MARGARINO, G.
Div. di Oncol. Chir. Instit. Nazion. per la Ricerca sul Cancro, Viale B.XV, I-16132 Genoa, Italy

MARGARIT, C.
Unidad Trasplante Hepatico, Hospital Vall d'Hebron, P. Vall d'Hebron 119-129, E-08035 Barcelona, Spain

MARTINEZ IBAÑEZ, V.
Ped. Surg. Dept., Hosp. Infantil Valle d'Hebron, E-08035 Barcelona, Spain

MARTUCCIELLO, G.
Univ. of Genoa "G. Gaslini" Inst. Genoa, Largo G. Gaslini, 5, I-16148 Genoa, Italy

MATTIOLI, G.
Univ. of Genoa "G. Gaslini" Inst. Genoa, Largo G. Gaslini, 5, I-16148 Genoa, Italy

MAU, H.
Kinderchir. Abt., St. Elisabethklinik Saarlouis, D-66740 Saarlouis, Federal Republic of Germany

MESZAROS, P.
Div. di Oncol. Chir. Instit. Nazion. per la Ricerca sul Cancro, Viale B.XV, I-16132 Genoa, Italy

MICCOLI, P.
Cattedra di Endocrinochir., Clin. Chir. dell' Univ. di Pisa, v. Roma 67, CAP 56100 Pisa, Italy

MIKAMI, T.
1st Dept. of Surg. Sapporo Med. Coll., S. 1, W. 16, Chuo-ku, Sapporo, 060 Japan

MOESCHL, P.
2nd Surg. Dept., Universität Wien, Spitalgasse 23, A-1090 Wien, Austria

MORESCO, L.
Clin. and Exp. Oncol. Inst. Univ. of Genoa, I-16132 Genoa, Italy

Morimoto, T.
2nd Dept. of Surg., Faculty of Med., Kyoto Univ., 54 Kawaramachi, Shogoin, Sakyo-ku, Kyoto 606 Japan

Mukaiya, M.
1st Dept. of Surg. Sapporo Med. Coll., S. 1, W. 16, Chuo-ku, Sapporo, 060 Japan

Murio, E.
H-P-B and Liver Transplant. Univ. Dept. of Surg. Hospital General Vall d'Hebron, Univ. Autónoma, E-08035 Barcelona, Spain

Oikawa, I.
1st Dept. of Surg. Sapporo Med. Coll., S. 1, W. 16, Chuo-ku, Sapporo, 060 Japan

Okazaki, A.
1st Dept. of Surg. Sapporo Med. Coll., S. 1, W. 16, Chuo-ku, Sapporo, 060 Japan

Oturandlar, D.
2nd Surg. Dept., Universität Wien, Spitalgasse 23, A-1090 Wien, Austria

Ozawa, K.
2nd Dept. of Surg., Faculty of Med., Kyoto Univ., 54 Kawaramachi, Shogoin, Sakyo-ku, Kyoto 606 Japan

Pechan, J.
2nd Dept. of Surg. Med. Faculty Comenius Univ., Bezrucova 5, CSRF-815 26 Bratislava

Peitz, U.
Medizinische Klinik, Elisabeth-Krankenhaus, Akademisches Lehrkrankenhaus, Universität Essen, Moltkestraße 61, D-45138 Essen, Federal Republic of Germany

Perez Martinez, Al.
Ped. Surg. Dept. Hosp. Infantil Valle d'Hebron, E-08035 Barcelona, Spain

Pretagostini, R.
II. Patol. Spec. Chir. Univ. di Roma "La Sapienza", I-00167 Rome, Italy

Puccini, M.
Cattedra di Endocrinochir., Clin. Chir. dell'Univ. di Pisa, v. Roma 67, CAP 56100 Pisa, Italy

Ricci, E.
Cattedra di Endocrinochir., Clin. Chir. dell'Univ. di Pisa, v. Roma 67, CAP 56100 Pisa, Italy

Rocca, M.
Exp. Surg. Dept. I.O.R., Univ. of Bologna, I-40136 Bologna, Italy

Rossi, M.
II. Patol. Spec. Chir. Univ. di Roma "La Sapienza",
I-00167 Rome, Italy

Roth, H.
Department of Pediatric Surgery, Universität Heidelberg,
Im Neuenheimer Feld 110, D-69121 Heidelberg,
Federal Republic of Germany

Sasaki, K.
1st Dept. of Surg., Sapporo Med. Coll., S.1, W.16, Chuo-ku,
Sapporo, 060 Japan

Scala, M.
Div. di Oncol. Chir. Instit. Nazion. per la Ricerca sul Cancro,
Viale B.XV, I-16132 Genoa, Italy

Schenone, G.
Div. di Oncol. Chir. Instit. Nazion. per la Ricerca sul Canero,
Viale B.XV, I-16132 Genoa, Italy

Schneider-Brown, H.
Kinderchirurgische Klinik, Städtisches Klinikum Karlsruhe,
Karl-Wilhelm-Straße 1, D-76131 Karlsruhe, Federal Republic
of Germany

Schnorrer, M.
2 nd Dept. of Surg. Med. Faculty Comenius Univ. Bezrucova 5,
CSRF-81526 Bratislava

Specht, U.
Kinderchirurgische Abteilung, St.-Elisabeth-Klinik,
D-66740 Saarlouis, Federal Republic of Germany

Schürmann, G.
Surgery Department, Universität Heidelberg, Im Neuenheimer
Feld 110, D-69120 Heidelberg, Federal Republic of Germany

Stipa, S.
Dept. of Surg., I°Instit. di Clin. Chir., Univ. of Rome,
"La Sapienza", I-00167 Rome, Italy

Tanaka, A.
2nd Dept. of Surg., Faculty of Med., Kyoto Univ., 54 Kawaramachi,
Shogoin, Sakyo-ku, Kyoto 606 Japan

Tanaka, K.
2nd Dept. of Surg., Faculty of Med., Kyoto Univ., 54 Kawaramachi,
Shogoin, Sakyo-ku, Kyoto 606 Japan

Tokunaga, Y.
2nd Dept. of Surg., Faculty of Med., Kyoto Univ., 54 Kawaramachi,
Shogoin, Sakyo-ku, Kyoto 606 Japan

Tomei, D.
Div. di Oncol. Chir. Instit. Nazion. per la Ricerca sul Cancro,
Viale B.XV, I-16132 Genoa, Italy

UEMOTO, S.
2nd Dept. of Surg., Faculty of Med., Kyoto Univ., 54 Kawaramachi, Shogoin, Sakyo-ku, Kyoto 606 Japan

URANÜS, S.
Dept. of Gen. Surg. Karl-Franzens-Universität, Auenbrugger Platz 15, A-8036 Graz, Austria

VALAYER, J.
Dept. de Péd., Univ. Paris Sud, CHU de Bicêtre, 78 Rue du Général Leclerc, F-94275 Kremlin Bicêtre, France

VECCHIO, C.
Div. di Oncol. Chir. Instit. Nazion. per la Ricerca sul Cancro, Viale B.XV, I-16132 Genoa, Italy

WACLAWICZEK, H. W.
1st Surg. Dept. LKA Salzburg, Müllner Hauptstr. 48, A-5020 Salzburg, Austria

WIECZOREK, M.
Medizinische Klinik, Elisabeth-Krankenhaus, Akademisches Lehrkrankenhaus, Universität Essen, Moltkestraße 61, D-45138 Essen, Federal Republic of Germany

WILLITAL, G. H.
Klinik f. Kinder- u. Neugeb.-Chir., Westfäl.-Wilhelms-Univ., Albert-Schweitzer-Str. 33, D-48149 Münster, Federal Republic of Germany

WIRTH, H.
Kinderchirurgische Klinik, Städtisches Klinikum Karlsruhe, Karl-Wilhelm-Straße 1, D-76131 Karlsruhe, Federal Republic of Germany

YAMAOKA, Y.
2nd Dept. of Surg., Faculty of Med., Kyoto Univ., 54 Kawaramachi, Shogoin, Sakyo-ku, Kyoto 606 Japan

YAMASIRO, K.
1st Dept. of Surg. Sapporo Med.Coll., S. 1, W. 16, Chuo-ku, Sapporo, 060 Japan

YANDZA, T.
Dept. de Péd., Univ. Paris Sud, CHU de Bicêtre, 78 Rue du Général Leclerc, F-94275 Kremlin Bicêtre, France

ZACHARIOU, Z.
Department of Pediatric Surgery, Universität Heidelberg, Im Neuenheimer Feld 110, D-69120 Heidelberg, Federal Republic of Germany

I. General and Abdominal Surgery

Experience with the Use of a Fibrin Sealant (Tissucol) in Liver Surgery

C. Margarit, J. Balsells, R. Charco, J. L. Lázaro, E. Murio, A. Edo, and I. Diaz

Abstract

We present our experience with the use of a fibrin sealant (Tissucol, Immuno, Vienna) applied to the raw surface of the liver after resection. During a 4-year period, 102 hepatic resections were performed in 100 patients. Hepatic tumors, particularly hepatocellular carcinoma in cirrhotic liver, were the main indication, followed by metastasic lesions from colorectal cancer. Almost half of the patients submitted to hepatic resection had liver cirrhosis and therefore had an increased risk of postoperative liver failure, coagulopathy and hemorrhage. Tissucol was applied after hepatic parenchymal division and hemostasis of the blood vessels and bile ducts had been achieved using ligatures and electrocautery. A collagen felt was also placed on the raw surface in 20 % of cases.

Postoperative mortality (9.8 %) and morbidity was low, considering the high percentage of cirrhotic patients. Liver failure was the principal cause of death. In conclusion, a very careful surgical technique and the application of Tissucol to seal off the raw surface of the liver avoided in most cases the complications of oozing and biliary leakage, which would lead to hemorrhage, abscess, sepsis, and consequently liver failure.

Introduction

We review the experience with liver resections during the 4-year period that our unit, dedicated to liver surgery and transplantation, has been active. The fibrin sealant (Tissucol, Immuno, Vienna) has been used in experimental and clinical liver transplantation, particularly in cases of reduced, segmental, or split grafts. We were able to demonstrate the perfect hemostasis achieved with a combination of Tissucol and collagen [1, 2] (Fig. 1). We followed the same principles in treating the raw surface of the liver after resection, particularly in cases of nonanatomical resections in cirrhotic patients.

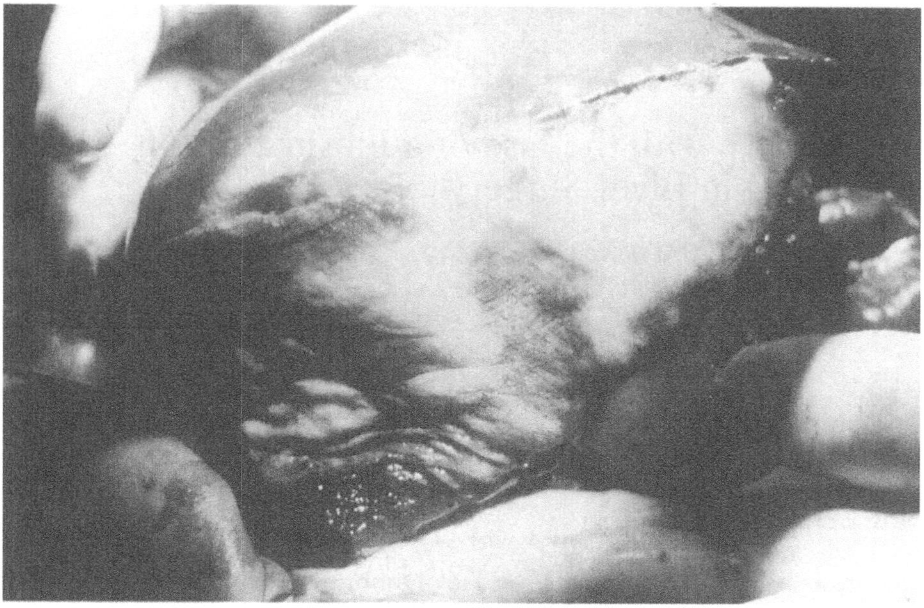

Fig. 1. Reduced-size liver graft after revascularization; perfect hemostasis with Tissucol and collagen

Materials

From 1988 to 1992, 102 hepatic resections in 100 patients were performed in our unit. Demographics and indications are shown in Table 1. The main indications for liver resection in our experience are hepatocellular carcinoma in cirrhotic liver, followed by metastases from colorectal cancer. As far as benign diseases are concerned, hemangiomas and hydatid cysts have been the most important groups. Nevertheless, in eight cases a preoperative diagnosis of possible malignant tumor was not confirmed in the final pathology report and those patients are included in the group of benign diseases.

Cirrhosis of the liver was present in 45 patients, and most of them had hepatocellular cancer. Only those cirrhotic patients with good liver function – groups A and B according to the Child-Pough classification – and presenting single and well-limited tumors were considered for resection.

Methods

The type of hepatic resections performed in this group of 100 patients are shown in Tables 2–4. Anatomical resections, i.e., hepatic resection following the lobar and segmental divisions of the liver, generally with vascular and biliar control at the porta hepatis, were performed in cases of malignant or benign tumors in normal livers, whereas nonanatomical resections were more often

Table 1. Demographics and indications for liver resection

Indications	Number of patients
Primary malignant tumors	49
Hepatocellular carcinoma	44
Hepatocellular carcinoma with liver cirrhosis	42
Cholangiocarcinoma	1
Embryonal sarcoma	1
Klatskin tumor	3
Secondary tumors: metastases	30
Colorectal cancer	23
Renal adenocarcinoma	2
Others	5
Trauma	2
Benign disease	21
Hemangioma	5
Hydatid cyst	6
Hepatic abscess	3
Regenerative nodule	3
Fibrous nodule	3
Caroli's disease	1

A total of 102 hepatic resections were performed in 100 patients (31 female, 69 male). Mean age, 56 ± 16 years (range, 14–81 years).

Table 2. Classification of hepatic resections

Type	Number of resections
Anatomical hepatic resections	59
Major hepatic resections	39
Right hepatectomy	23
Extended right hepatectomy	5
Left hepatectomy	8
Extended left hepatectomy	3
Minor hepatic resections	19
Segmentectomies	
Nonanatomical hepatic resections	43

Table 3. Type of hepatic resections regarding liver function

	Anatomical (%)	Nonanatomical (%)
Cirrhosis	31	69
Normal	76	23

Table 4. Use of Tissucol and Collagen

	Tissucol (%)	Collagen (%)
Total	61	23
Cirrhosis	86	50
Normal		
Malignant	35	–
Benign	50	–

performed in cases of tumors appearing in cirrhotic livers (Fig. 2). In those cases, intraoperative ultrasound examination was very useful to localize the tumor, making feasible its radical resection while preserving as much functional liver parenchyma as possible to avoid postoperative liver failure.

Frequently, additional operative procedures were performed: biliary operations such as radical resection of the extrahepatic biliary tree in Klatskin tumors or biliary exploration and drainage in hydatid cysts with biliary fistulas. Resection of the primary tumor along with the liver metastases was indicated in eight cases. In two cases a hepatocellular carcinoma was discovered on ultrasound examination of the liver after rupture of esophageal varices. A portacaval shunt and resection of the hepatoma was performed.

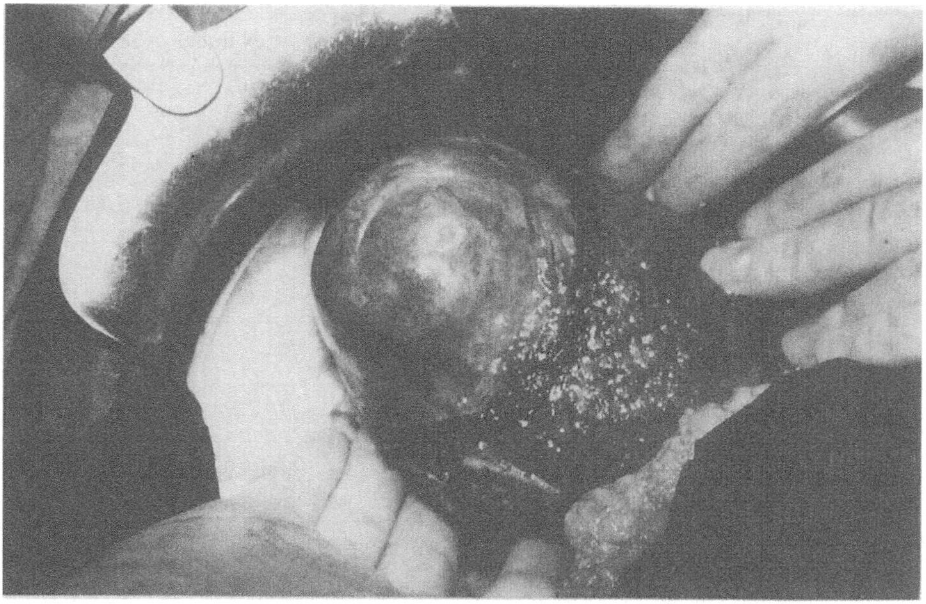

Fig. 2. Hepatocellular cancer in cirrhotic liver; limits of resection after ultrasound exploration

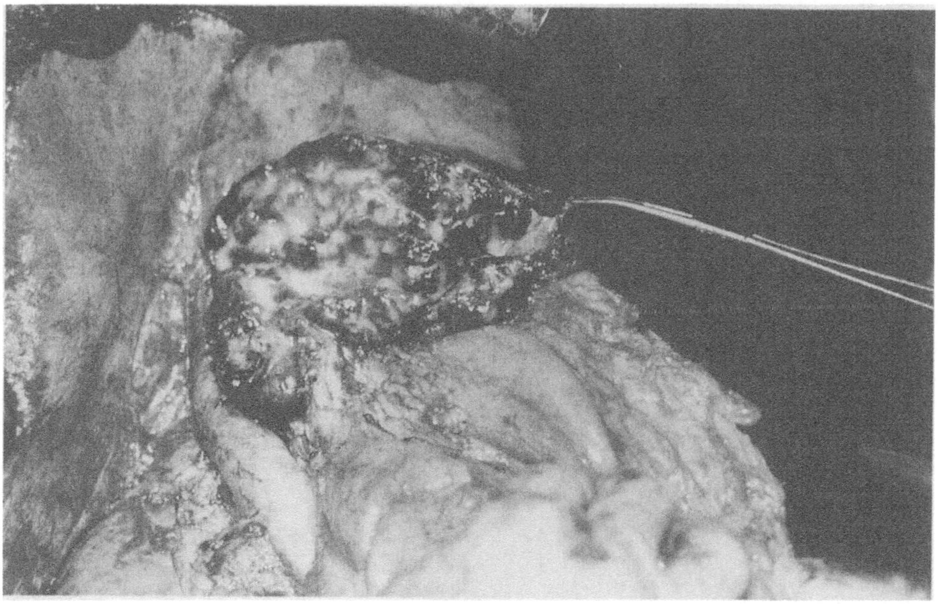

Fig. 3. Tissucol on the raw surface after extended right hepatectomy

Hemostatic Methods

The liver parenchyma was divided using a combination of electrocautery and Kelly fracture technique. The ultrasound dissector was used in a few cases. All vessels and biliar ducts were ligated. In 40 % of the cases, a Pringle maneuver was used during a mean time of 20 min. This technique diminished blood loss, particularly in nonanatomical resections in cirrhotic patients. Once the liver resection had been completed, extra time was dedicated to completing the hemostasis of the main bleeders. Finally, Tissucol was applied to the raw surface in 60 % of the cases (Fig. 3). A collagen felt was added in 23 hepatectomies in cirrhotic livers (Fig. 4).

Results

Operative mortality was 9.8 %, mainly due to liver failure in cases of cirrhosis. An increased operative mortality was found in the groups with hepatocellular carcinoma in cirrhotic liver, Klatskin tumors, and hepatic trauma (Table 5). Cause of death was liver failure in four cases, hemorrhage and liver failure in one case, pulmonary embolism in one case, mesenteric infarct in one case, septic shock in two cases, and multiorgan failure in one case. As far as postoperative complications were concerned, four patients presented with hemorrhage, but only one had to be reoperated. Biliary fistulas were observed in

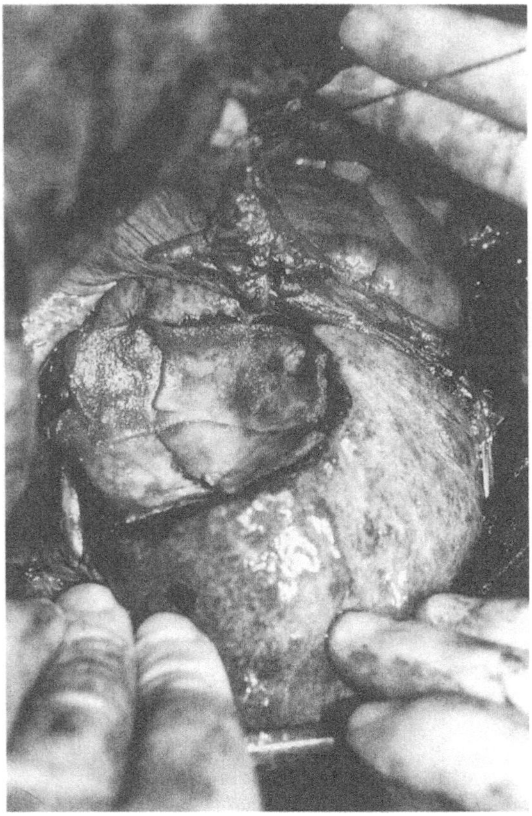

Fig. 4. Tissucol and collagen after nonanatomical resection of hepatocellular cancer in cirrhosis

eight cases, and half of them needed another operation. Hepatic dysfunction presenting as ascites and jaundice was quite common in cirrhotic patients; there were two cases each of wound infection, subphrenic abscess, and ascites and 13 cases of liver insufficiency.

Table 5. Results of hepatic resections. Postoperative mortality

Indication	*n*	Postoperative mortality	
		n	%
Hepatoma and cirrhosis	42	6	14.3
Secondary tumors	30	1	3.3
Klatskin tumors	3	2	66.6
Trauma	2	1	50.0
Benign diseases	21	0	0.0
Total	102	10	9.9

Discussion

In the past two decades there has been a revolution in liver surgery. The major contributions to the striking improvement in the results of liver resections have been the definition of the anatomy of the liver and consequently of the principles of anatomic and nonanatomic resections [3, 4] and the enormous advances in imaging techniques. Routine examination of populations at risk has made possible the early diagnosis of liver tumors such as hepatocellular carcinoma in cirrhotic liver or metastatic lesions, with the result that an increased number of patients are being referred for resection at early stages. The application of intraoperative ultrasound examination allows us to perform a radical tumor excision avoiding large hepatectomies, which may result in liver failure in the case of cirrhosis [5]. The liver is the most vascularized organ of the body; it has a double blood supply through the portal vein and hepatic artery. One third of the blood volume circulates through the liver. Massive hemorrhage and patient exsanguination is the worst operative complication of liver surgery. The surgeon's experience and his knowledge of anatomy is vital to perform a lobar or segmental anatomical resection with vascular control without undue blood loss. The Pringle maneuver is recommended in cases of nonanatomical resections in order to minimize blood loss during the hepatectomy. By means of careful, patient division of the liver parenchyma with the fingers, Kelly fracture technique, or the aid of the ultrasound dissector, all the blood vessels and bile ducts must be ligated. However, some oozing is always present and electrocautery, infrared, or argon coagulator can then be used. Postoperative liver dysfunction and failure manifests itself as coagulopathy and ascites. Cirrhotic patients and those submitted to major liver resections as extended right or left hemihepatectomies are more prone to develop those complications [6–8]. Postoperative hemorrhage and bile leakage are very dangerous complications which lead to formation of subphrenic abscesses, infection of ascitis, sepsis, and further deterioration of liver function, resulting in liver failure and death. In these cases, a complete seal of the raw surface is mandatory and it is achieved in our experience with the use of fibrin sealant with or without collagen.

We were able to demonstrate in this large series of high-risk patients submitted to hepatic resection a very low incidence of hemorrhagic complications and mortality following these principles.

References

1. Margarit C, Martinez-Ibáñez V, Lloret J et al. (1987) Segmental liver transplantation in pigs: use of a fibrin sealant and collagen as hemostatic agents. Transplant Proc. XIX: 3835–3837
2. Margarit C, Martinez-Ibáñez V, Lloret J et al. (1988) Experimental and clinical reduced-size orthotopic liver transplantation: a new method for securing hemostasis. Transplant Proc XX: 546–547
3. Couinaud C (1957) Etudes anatomiques et chirurgicales. Masson, Paris.

4. Bismuth H, Sherlock D J (1990) Revolution in liver surgery. Gastroenterol Hepatol [Suppl]. 1: 95–109
5. Bismuth H, Castaign D, Garden J (1987) The use of operative ultrasound in surgery of primary liver tumours. World J Surg 11: 610–614
6. Iwatsuki S, Starzl T E (1988) Personal experience with 411 hepatic resections. Ann Surg 208: 421–434
7. Franco D, Capussotti L, Smadja C et al. (1990) Resection of hepatocellular carcinomas. Results in 72 European patients with cirrhosis. Gastroenterology 98: 733–738
8. Margarit C, Balsells J, Lázaro JL et al. (1991) Resección de hepatocarcinomas en hígado cirrótico. Indicaciones, técnica y resultados. Cirug Esp 49: 405–410

Fibrin Sealing of the Cut Surface of Liver Grafts in Partial Liver Transplantation with Living Related Donors

K. Tanaka, Y. Tokunaga, S. Uemoto, T. Morimoto, A. Tanaka, Y. Yamaoka, and K. Ozawa

Abstract

One of the key issues in liver transplantation with living related donors (LRLT) is to control bleeding and bile leakage from the cut surface of the partial liver graft. For this purpose we covered the cut surface of the liver with fibrin sealant. From June 1990 to December 1992, we performed a series of 50 LRLT on children with end-stage liver disease, with the informed consent of their parents and the approval of the Ethics Committee of Kyoto University. In the donor, the cutting plane of liver resection was determined preoperatively based on the size and the vascular structure of the liver. Procurement of the partial liver graft was performed without vascular clamping and without graft manipulation to maintain graft viability. The hepatic parenchyma was transected with an ultrasonic aspirator, bipolar electrocautery, and elaborate ligation or suture ligation of the blood vessels. At the "back table", the blood vessels were prepared for smooth and prompt reconstruction and fibrin glue was sprayed on the dried cut surface using compressed air. Actuarial recipient survival rate was 90 % (37 out of 41) in elective cases and 67 % (six out of nine) in urgent cases. No bleeding or biliary leakage was observed on the cut surface throughout the operation or during the postoperative phase in any of the cases thus far. No definite puric discharge from the graft cut surface was observed at laparotomy for surgical complications after transplantation. Our initial experiences of liver transplantation involving living related donors indicated that fibrin sealant was effective in securing hemostasis and preventing bile leakage after elaborate ligation of the vessels and bile ducts in the cut surface.

Introduction

A number of innovative new technical devices introduced at each phase of the surgical procedures contributed to the overall success of our series of liver transplantation with living related donors (LRLT). They consisted of: (a) graft procurement without blood vessel clamping and without graft manipulation; (b) preoperative evaluation of anatomical variation of the hepatic and portal veins scheduled for reconstruction; and (c) microsurgical anastomosis of the hepatic artery [10, 15–18]. Complete hemostasis of the cut surface of the partial liver graft was another development that helped to make LRLT clinically feasible.

In this report, we present the surgical procedures of the graft procurement in living related donors, including the "back table" operation, and evaluate the effects of fibrin glue on hemostasis of the cut surface in terms of postoperative complications.

Materials and Methods

From June 1990 to December 1992, we preformed a series of 50 LRLT on children with end-stage liver disease, with the informed consent of their parents and the approval of the Ethics Committee of Kyoto University [12].

The plane of liver resection was determined preoperatively on the basis of donor liver volumetry using computed tomography. Anatomical variations and sizes of the vascular structures in individuals were assessed by ultrasonography (Toshiba SSA-270A; Toshiba, Tokyo) and magnetic resonance imaging (Sigma; GE Medical Systems, Milwaukee). According to the results of graft/recipient size matching, either a left lateral segmentectomy (S2+S3), left lateral segmentectomy with part of segment 4 (S2+S3+partial S4), or left lobectomy (S2+S3+S4) was performed [17] (Fig. 1).

After two rows of mattress sutures with 3-0 polypropylene (Prolene) were installed parallel to the line of transection, the hepatic parenchyma was incised between the two rows of suture using ultrasonic aspirator (CUSA; Cavitron, Stanford, CA). The clearly exposed vessels were either ligated or suture-ligated, while fibrous connecting tissues of the glissonian branches and tiny vessels were coagulated by a newly devised bipolar electrocautery equipped with a saline drip system [17].

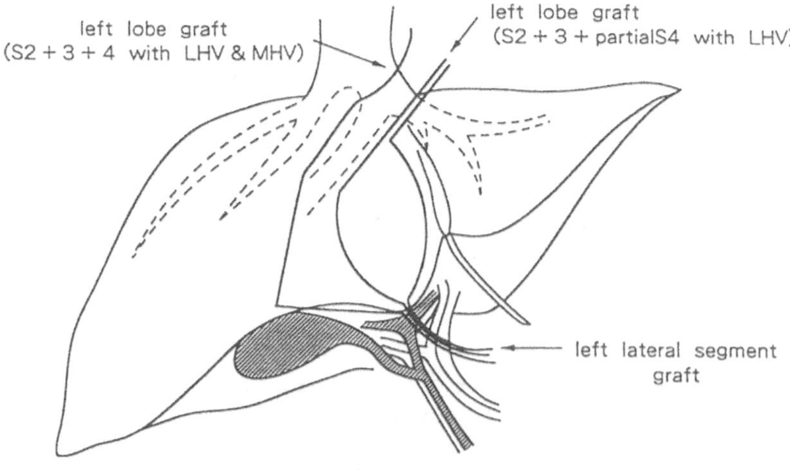

Fig. 1. The plane of liver resection was determined on the basis of donor liver volumetry and graft/recipient size matching using computed tomography. *S*, segment; *MHV*, middle hepatic vein; *LHV*, left hepatic vein

After the division of the parenchyma was completed, the medial branch of the middle hepatic vein was dissected and the right side of the vein was separated from the parenchyma down to the junction of the left hepatic vein. Small holes in the vein wall were suture-ligated with 6-0 Prolene. The triangular ligament and the hepatogastric ligament were divided and resected from the liver at this time. Extra care must be taken to ensure the blood flow to the bile duct. Although the hepatic artery and the portal vein were isolated from the Glisson's sheath, the sheath around the bile duct was left undisturbed so as to maintain the blood flow to the biliary system. The bile duct can then be severed a little to the left of the bifurcation with sharp incision. The hole created in the main bile duct was interrupted-sutured with 7-0 Prolene so as not to constrict the passage.

After the artery and hepatic vein were severed with sharp incision, the isolated liver graft was perfused in situ via the cannula inserted into the portal vein. The perfusate initially consisted of 200 ml chilled (4 °C) lactated Ringer's solution containing 400 units heparin and was later switched to 4 °C UW solution (600–1000 ml). The graft was then transported to the "back table" and placed in a specially designed basin filled with University of Wisconsin (UW) solution. The bottom of the basin was placed on ice to maintain the temperature of the solution below 4 °C.

At the back table, the hepatic vein and portal vein of the graft were prepared for smooth and prompt venous anastomosis. After removing the solution and drying the cut surface with sterile gauze, the cut surface was sprayed with thin film of fibrin glue (5 ml Tisseel; Immuno, Vienna) using compressed air at a rate of 5–10 l/min (Tissomat Duploject Spray; Immuno, Vienna) to secure hemostasis. The orifices of the blood vessels and bile duct were protected from the glue by covering them with the operator's fingers (Fig. 2).

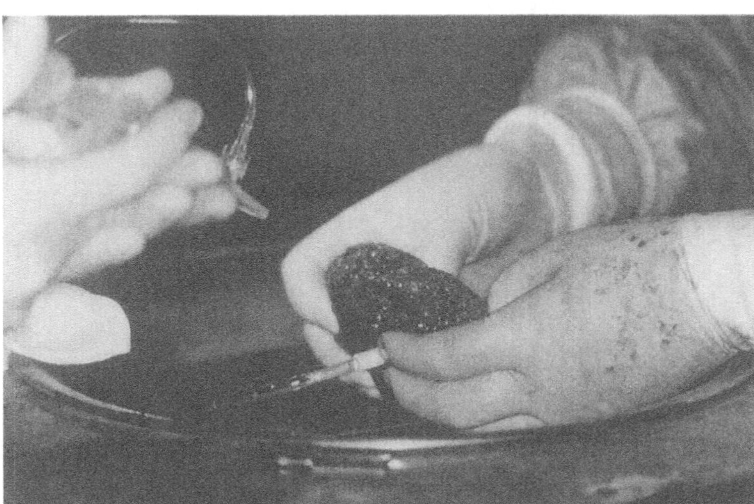

Fig. 2. Fibrin glue is sprayed on the cut surface of the partial liver graft using compressed air. The orifice of the blood vessels and bile duct are protected from the glue sealant

Results

All donors had normal liver function and no history of liver disease. Blood loss during procurement was always less than 500 g and no blood transfusion was needed in any of the cases. They were discharged from the hospital at 10–17 (mean, 11.6) days after surgery without any complications which required surgical intervention and were able to return to normal life. Actuarial recipient survival rate was 90 % (37 out of 41) in elective cases and 67 % (six out of nine) in urgent cases. Seven recipients died in spite of functioning grafts due to extrahepatic complications, including one accidental aspiration asphyxia, two cardiac insufficiencies, two multiple organ failures, one *Candida* infection, and one lymphoproliferative disorder.

Blood loss in the recipient operations ranged from 13 to 933 (mean, 180) g/kg body weight (Fig. 3). At reperfusion of the graft, we have not experienced blood loss from the cut surface thus far. However, bile oozing on the cut surface was observed in two of the 50 cases, requiring suture ligation of minute holes in the small branch of the bile duct with 6-0 Prolene. Peritoneal hemorrhage occurred in eight cases as a result of bleeding at the vascular anastomosis, dissected surface of the intestine, and/or unidentified origin, and biliary leakage developed in six cases, occurring in most cases from pinhole perforations at the closed jejunal stump used previously for jejunostomy. However, no bleeding or biliary leakage was observed on the cut surface throughout the operation (Fig. 4) or during the postoperative phase in any of the cases.

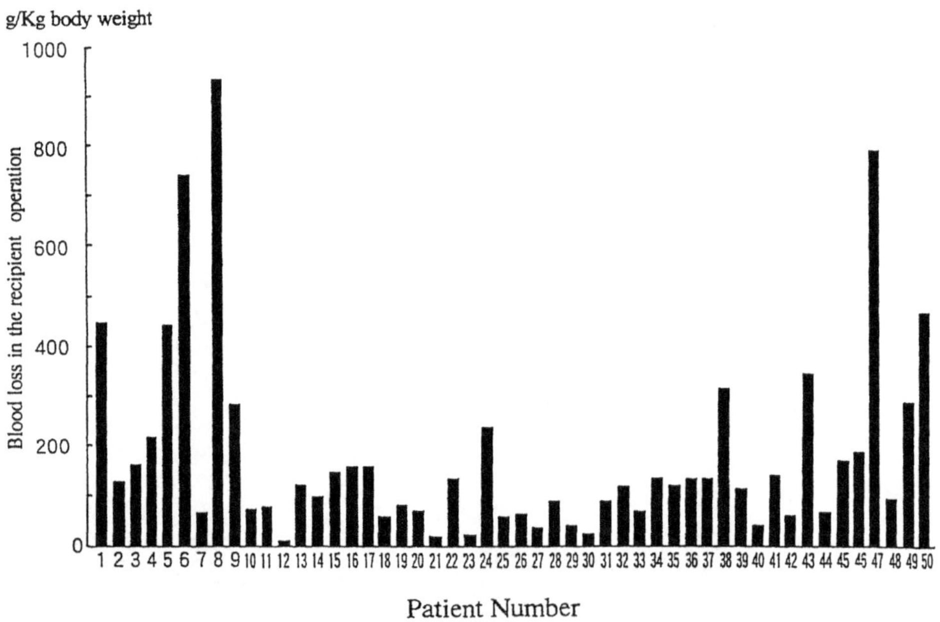

Fig. 3. Blood loss in recipient operations decreased along with the learning curve except for complicated cases. No bleeding from the cut surface has been experienced in any case thus far

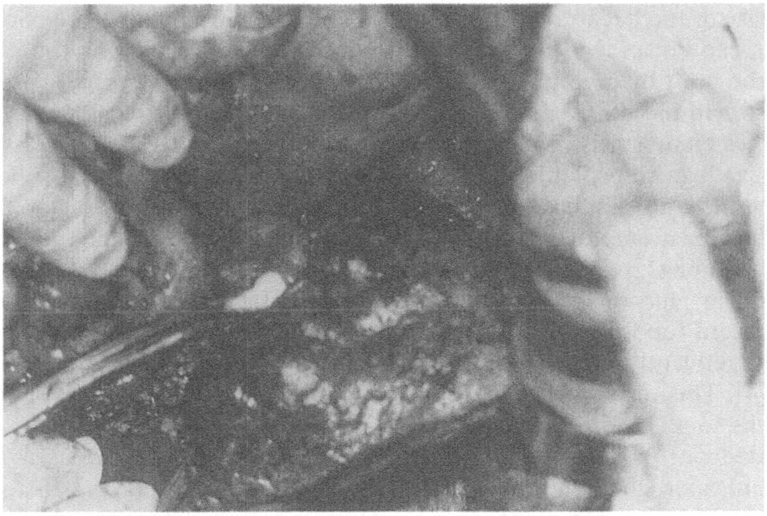

Fig. 4. Cut surface of the partial liver graft at the end of operation. No bleeding and biliary leakage occurred during the operation in any of the cases

Infectious complication due to bacteria occurred in seven cases (one cholangitis, one wound infection, two cases of generalized peritonitis, and three of regional peritonitis). They were associated with surgical complications such as biliary leakage, bilioenteric anastomotic stenosis, or intestinal perforation. All of them were treated successfully by antibiotics and surgical intervention including peritoneal drainage, percutaneous transhepatic bile duct dilatation, or creation of ileostomy. There has been no definite puric discharge from the cut surface observed at laparotomy for surgical complications.

Discussion

Complete hemostasis and prevention of bile leakage at the cut surface of the graft and the remnant donor liver as well as the graft viability are basic desiderata for successful outcome in LRLT. Our strategies for hemostasis and prevention of biliary leakage are: (a) elaborate ligation of the blood vessels and electrocoagulation of the fibrous tissue using bipolar electrocautery equipped with a saline drip system; (b) covering of almost the entire cut surface with fibrin glue; (c) suture ligation of tiny holes in the bile duct in the cut surface; and (d) maintenance of the arterioles in Glisson's sheath to avoid ischemic damage to the biliary system. The strategies to maintain graft viability are harvesting without blood vessel clamping and without graft manipulation. We prefer to use fibrin glue at the back table rather than in situ on the donor, since the cut surface can be exposed much better ex situ without any kinking of the graft blood vessels. Also, since the graft hepatic vein should be prepared for smooth and prompt anastomosis and the graft volume should be adjusted to the recipient size at the back table, fibrin glue should be employed at the back table, where it can be sprayed on the dried surface without disturbing the blood supply to the graft by manipulating it in situ. Ideally, compressed air should be used to spread the fibrin glue in a thin, even film.

Hemostasis of the graft cut surface has been also a major issue in reduced-size liver transplantation. Bismuth covered the cut surface of the reduced liver graft in his first case with a gelatin-resorcin-formaldehyde glue [1]. Fibrin glue has been employed in most transplant institutes all over the world [3, 7, 13], including a relatively large series by Otte et al. [6, 11]. However, the efficacy of fibrin glue on hemostasis of the cut surface has seldom been discussed. A recent report by Esquivel et al. reported that the transfusion requirement was significantly greater in reduced-size transplant than in whole liver transplant [4]. This difference is perhaps due to the difficulty in identifying and ligating the small blood vessels of the cut surface, since hepatic resection is usually carried out in the exsanguinated liver following flush perfusion.These findings indicated that without ligation of the blood vessel, satisfactory hemostasis would be hard to obtain solely by fibrin sealant. Thus, one should bear in mind that fibrin glue is always to be used as a final and additional material to secure the surgical hemostasis rather than the primary maneuver to control bleeding from the cut surface, although it may be a potentially useful material for sutureless anastomosis and hemostasis in various experimental animals [2, 5]. The primary procedure is always elaborate ligation of the blood vessels and coagulation of the connective tissue by bipolar cautery.

Fibrin glue has been employed in various surgical fields on the assumption that it causes little foreign body reaction [2,5, 8]. In a study on experimentally produced hepatic injuries in dogs, Kram et al. demonstrated that hemostasis was achieved without any intra-abdominal infection or abscess formation as evidenced in postoperative liver specimens [9]. On the other hand, a recent study on colonic perforation in rats indicated a possible granulation by fibrin glue in the repair process of perforation [14]. Although there have been controversial findings in experimental animals, no infectious and foreign body reactions have been observed thus far in the fibrin-sealed cut surface of the liver graft in our clinical series.

Acknowledgement
This work was supported in part by grants from the Scientific Research Fund of the Ministry of Education and by a Grant-in-Aid for Cancer Research from the Ministry of Health and Welfare, Japan.

References

1. Bismuth H, Houssin D (1984) Reduced-sized orthotopic liver graft in hepatic transplantation in children. Surgery 95: 367–370
2. Blair GK, Castner P, Tayler G, Newman D, Santoso B (1988) Espophageal atresia – a rabbit model to study anastomotic healing and the use of tissue adhesive fibrin sealant. J Pediatr Surg 23: 740–743
3. Broelsch CE, Whitington PF, Emond JC et al. (1992) Liver transplantation in children from living related donors. Ann Surg 214: 428–439

4. Esquivel CO, Nakazato P, Cox K, Concepcion W, Berquist W, Russell TR (1991) The impact of liver reduction in pediatric liver transplantation, Arch Surg 126: 1278–1286
5. Haukipuro KA, Hulkko OA, Alavaikko MJ, Laitinen ST (1988) Sutureless colon anastomosis with fibrin glue in the rat. Dis Colon Rectum 31: 601–604
6. Hemptinne B, de Ville de Goyet J, Kesten PJ, Otte JB (1987) Volume reduction of the liver graft before orthotopic transplantation: report of a clinical experience in 11 cases. Transplant Proc 19: 3317–3322
7. Kalayoglu M, D'Allessandro AM, Sollinger HW, Hoffman RM, Pirsch JD, Belzer RO (1990) Experience with reduced-size liver transplantation. Surg Gynec Obstet 171: 139–147
8. Karacsonyi S, Farkas G, Karacsonyi M, Bajusz H, Olah T (1986) Survey of liver regeneration following liver resection by application of fibrin sealant. Schlag G, Redl H (eds) Fibrin-sealant in operative medicine, general surgery and abdominal surgery, vol 6 Springer, Berlin Heidelberg New York, pp 85–90
9. Kram HB, Reuben BI, Fleming AW, Shoemaker WC (1988) Use of fibrin glue in hepatic trauma. J Trauma 28: 1195–1201
10. Mori K, Nagata I, Yamagata S et al. (1992). The introduction of microvascular surgery to hepatic artery reconstruction in living donor liver transplantation: its surgical advantages compared to conventional procedures. Transplantation 52: 263–268
11. Otte JB, de Ville de Goyet J, Sokal E et al. (1990) Size reduction of the donor liver is a safe way to alleviate the shortage of size-matched organs in pediatric liver transplantation. Ann Surg 211: 146–157
12. Ozawa K, Uemoto S, Tanaka K et al. (1992) An appraisal of pediatric liver transplantation from living relatives: initial clinical experiences in 20 pediatric liver transplantations from living relatives as donors. Ann Surg 216: 547–553
13. Ringe B, Pichlmayr R, Burdelski M (1988) A new technique of hepatic vein reconstruction in partial liver transplantation. Transplant Int 1: 30–35
14. Sanal M, Dogruyol H, Gurpinar A, Yerci O (1992) Does fibrin glue cause foreign body reactions? Eur J Pediatr Surg 2: 285–286
15. Tanaka K, Uemoto S, Tokunaga Y et al. Surgical techniques and innovations in living related liver transplantation. Ann Surg (in press)
16. Tokunaga Y, Tanaka K, Yamaoka Y et al. Portal vein graft in living related liver transplantation. Surg Gynec Obstet (in press)
17. Yamaoka Y, Ozawa K, Tanaka K et al. (1991) New devices for harvesting a hepatic graft from a living donor. Transplantation 52: 157–160
18. Yamaguchi T, Yamaoka Y, Mori K et al. Hepatic vein reconstruction of the graft in partial liver transplantation from living donor: surgical procedures relating to their anatomical variations. Surgery (in press)

Preoperative Portal Vein Embolization with Fibrin Sealant for Hepatocellular Carcinoma

S. Kubo, H. Kinoshita, and K. Hirohashi

Abstract

Liver resection is the most effective therapy for hepatocellular carcinoma (HCC), but associated chronic liver diseases such as cirrhosis of the liver often limit its use. We started to use portal vein embolization (PVE) with an adhesive mixture of fibrin as an adjuvant therapy to improve the outcome of surgical treatment. We investigated the clinical course after PVE and operative specimens in which PVE had been done. PVE strengthened the anticancer effect of transcatheter arterial embolization (TAE). PVE causes regeneration of the nonembolized lobe and atrophy of the embolized lobe, which extends the surgical indications for patients with HCC and makes surgery safer if the patients have cirrhosis. Nonrecurrence survival rates in the patients in whom preoperative PVE had been done tended to be better than in the patients without this treatment. PVE seems to be useful as preparation for surgery and as one therapy for unresectable HCC, usually to be done together with other treatments.

Introduction

The prognosis of hepatocellular carcinoma (HCC) has been improved by new surgical procedures and current preoperative and postoperative management, but the prognosis of advanced HCC, with portal invasion or associated chronic liver diseases, is still poor. About 80 % of Japanese patients with HCC have cirrhosis of the liver [1], which limits the surgical indications and can give rise to acute hepatic failure after surgery. In addition, portal invasion such as portal thrombus is often found even if the tumor is small [2]; invasion is one of the most important prognostic factors for HCC [1, 3, 4].

To improve the long-term survival rate of patients with HCC, we tried transcatheter arterial embolization (TAE) before liver resection. However, TAE had little if any effect on portal invasion and small intrahepatic metastases [5]. The outcome of patients treated by TAE and liver resection was not much better than that of those undergoing liver resection alone [6].

We devised a method to embolize the portal vein by percutaneous transhepatic portal vein catheterization and performed percutaneous transhepatic portal vein embolization (PVE) for its anticancer effects against HCC (the main tumor, portal invasion, and intrahepatic metastases) and to extend the surgical indications for HCC with cirrhosis of the liver [6, 7].

In this paper, we describe the technique of this procedure and report the results of treatment with PVE for this disease.

Materials and Methods

Our subjects were 54 patients with HCC scheduled for liver resection. Fifty patients were men and the other four were women. They were aged from 37 to 72 years old. Forty patients had cirrhosis of the liver, and TAE was done before PVE in 50 of the 54 patients.

We investigated the changes in the clinical course after PVE. We also studied the anticancer effects of PVE (with TAE earlier) in operative specimens, comparing the results with those in patients who underwent TAE and liver resection without PVE. The outcomes in the three groups (group N, liver resection only; group A, TAE and liver resection; group AP, TAE, PVE, and liver resection) were compared.

PVE was done as follows. A portal branch in the noncancerous area was punctured under sonographic guidance by the Seldinger method. Portography with a 5.5-F catheter was done with vertical and horizontal beams, serving both to clarify the ramifications of the intrahepatic portal veins and to detect portal invasion such as by portal thrombi. The branch (or branches) to be embolized (usually that supplying the area to be resected) was identified. Then, through a 6.5-F catheter introducer, a 6.0-F double-lumen balloon catheter was introduced into the branch of the portal vein. The balloon was inflated and embolic materials, such as an adhesive mixture of fibrin (6.4% fibrinogen mixed with an equal volume of 5 units thrombin per milliliter water) with iodized oil (Lipiodol) added to give radiopacity, were injected under fluoroscopic control. After embolization, the balloon catheter was removed and the part of the portal vein punctured was identified. Then, the puncture wound of the liver was blocked with gelatin sponge through the lumen of the introducer to prevent intraperitoneal bleeding.

Usually, TAE was done by the method of Yamada et al. [8], PVE was done about 2 weeks later, and liver resection was done 2 or 3 weeks after the PVE.

Abdominal X-ray films are taken after PVE so that the completeness of the embolization and the changes after PVE can be checked (Fig. 1) [9].

Results

Clinical Course after Portal Vein Embolization

Immediately after PVE, portal pressure increased by 20–40 mm H_2O. Most patients had abdominal discomfort or pain and fever after PVE. These side effects were mild and transitory. There was often a transitory rise in the leukocyte count. Aspartate aminotransferase (AST) and alanine aminotransferase (ALT)

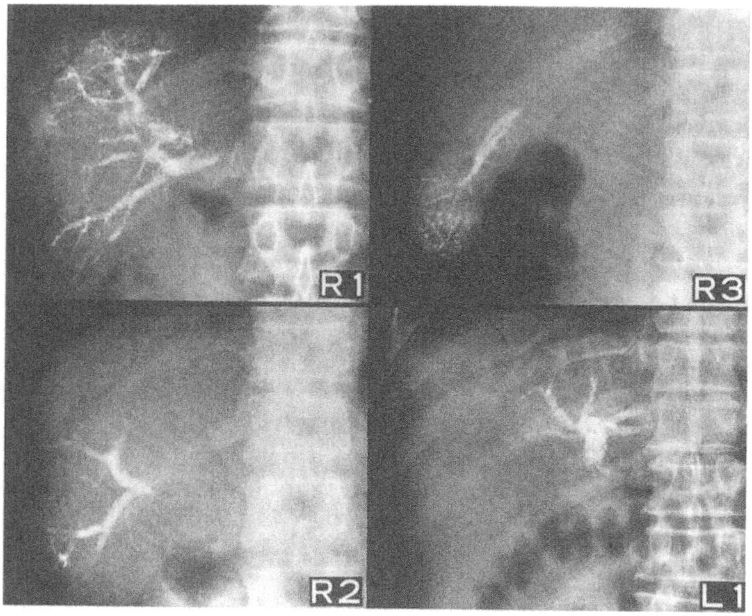

Fig. 1. Pictures taken during portal vein embolization (PVE). Radiopaque areas show an embolus in the portal vein. The portal branches embolized are the left first branch (L1), the right first branch (R1), the right second branch (R2), and a more peripheral branch (R3)

increased in almost all patients, but the increases were transitory. All three values decreased within 2 weeks after PVE. In patients who underwent embolization of the right first branch of the portal vein, computed tomograms taken before and after PVE were compared. The volume of the nonembolized area (the left lobe) increased greatly (Fig. 2). The changes in volume of the lobes in patients grouped by the area of the embolization were compared. After PVE, the embolized lobe tended to become smaller, and the lobe not embolized tended to become larger. The increase in volume of the nonembolized area was the largest in the patients who underwent embolization of the right first branch of the portal vein.

At laparotomy, the appearance of the area affected by PVE varied depending on the state of embolization of the portal branch and on recanalization of the occluded artery. The embolized area was dark red, which produced a line of demarcation between the embolized and the nonembolized part of the liver. These portal branches were filled with the embolic material.

Anticancer Effect of Portal Vein Embolization Seen by Histology

A histological study was done of the cancerous region of the segment occluded by TAE plus PVE (group AP). We also examined these regions after TAE alone (group A) in 129 other patients not part of the PVE study. In our 54 sub-

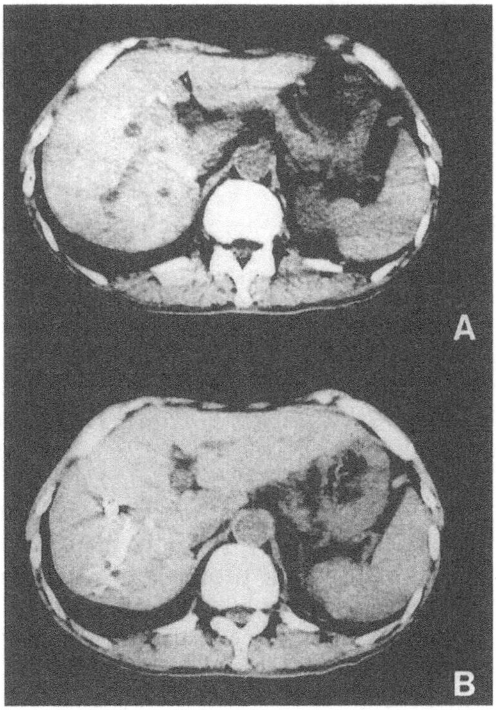

Fig. 2 A, B. Computed tomograms before (A) 2 weeks after (B) portal vein embolization (PVE). The left lobe is larger than before

jects in group AP, the main tumors in 25 of the patients (46 %) were completely necrotic. In the 129 patients in group A, 48 (37 %) main tumors were completely necrotic (Table 1). In 20 of the 28 (71 %) subjects found to have intrahepatic metastases in group AP, we found one or more of the metastases to be necrotic. In only 14 of the 36 (39 %) patients in group A we found to have metastases was one or more of the metastases necrotic. A portal thrombus was found in 11 patients in group AP. In seven (64 %), almost all of the thrombus cells we examined were necrotic. In six of 25 (24 %) portal thrombi found in group A, necrosis was seen. Thus, the histological findings in group AP were better than those in group A (Table 2).

Table 1. Anticancer effects of transcatheter arterial embolization (TAE) only or TAE plus portal vein embolization (PVE) on main tumors

Necrotic rate	Procedure			
	TAE only		TAE plus PVE	
(%)	*(n)*	(%)	*(n)*	(%)
100	48	37	25	46
50–90	47	36	20	37
1–49	23	18	6	11
0	11	9	3	6
Total –	129	100	54	100

Table 2. Anticancer effects of transcatheter arterial embolization (TAE) only or TAE plus portal vein embolization (PVE) on intrahepatic metastases and portal thrombi

Anticancer effect	Procedure					
	TAE only			TAE plus PVE		
	Positive effect *(n)*	Total *(n)*	(%)	Positive effect *(n)*	Total *(n)*	(%)
Intrahepatic metastasis	14	36	39	20	28	71
Portal thrombus	6	25	24	7	11	64

Extended Surgical Indications and Increased Safety of Liver Resection

To find whether PVE can extend surgical indications and increase the safety of liver resection, we studied the postoperative course after major liver resection, i.e., right lobectomy with or without PVE. Serum levels of AST, ALT, and total bilirubin (T-bil) and prothrombin time were measured. There was no significant difference in ALT or T-bil between these two groups, but the changes in AST and prothrombin time in the patients with PVE were significantly smaller than in the patients without PVE.

In the patients with PVE, the volume of the left (nonembolized) lobe increased after PVE and liver resection. However, the extent of increase in the volume of the left lobe from the beginning of treatment to 4 weeks after surgery in the patients with PVE was similar to that in the patients without PVE. These results mean that PVE causes the regeneration of the left lobe to occur in two stages.

Survival Rate

The longest time we have monitored a patient who underwent resection after TAE plus PVE is now 9.5 years. We calculated the nonrecurrence survival rates, because the usual survival rate is affected by the treatment after the detection of recurrence after the first operation. We compared the nonrecurrence survival rates in groups AP, A, and N (liver resection only) retrospectively. There was no difference in underlying liver function in these three groups. The stage of the tumor (according to the UICC classification [10]) in group AP tended to be more advanced than in the other groups. The nonrecurrence survival rate in group AP tended to be better then in the other groups (Fig. 3). Because treatment including PVE was more effective for portal thrombi, we studied the outcome of eight patients who had tumor thrombi in the first branch of the portal vein. Only two of these patients, both in group AP, survived long. In such patients, the tumor thrombi in the portal vein were covered by the embolic material (Fig. 4).

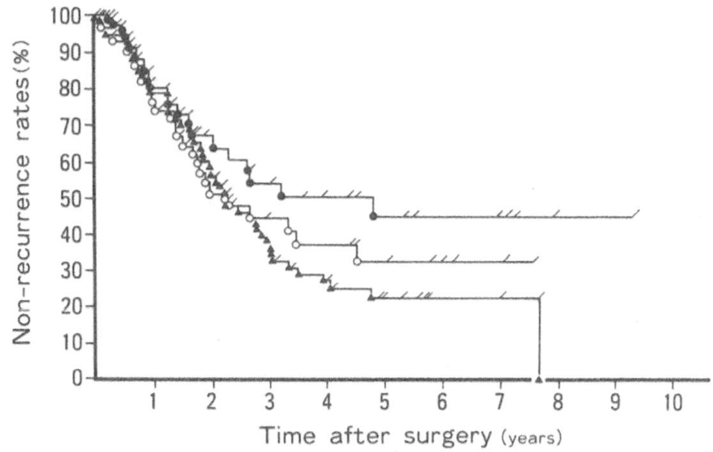

Fig. 3. Nonrecurrence survival rates with different treatments. *Solid circles*, transcatheter arterial embolization (TAE) plus portal vein embolization (PVE) plus resection; *open circles*, TAE plus resection; *triangles* resection only

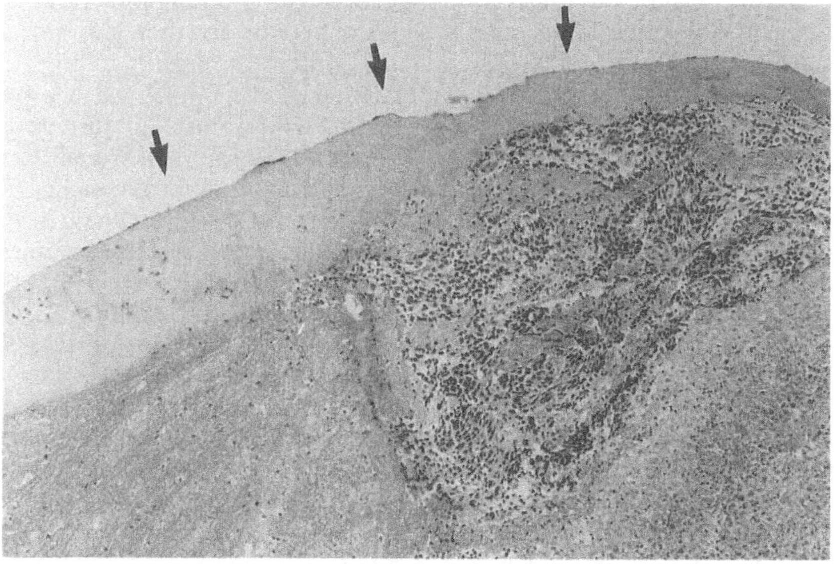

Fig. 4. Histological findings after portal vein embolization (PVE) in a patient with a portal thrombus in the first branch of the portal vein. The portal thrombus is covered by embolic material (*arrows*)

Discussion

Recently, small hepatocellular carcinomas have been discovered more frequently because of improvements in screening procedures and in medical imaging. However, even small tumors often progress to portal invasion. Since TAE is generally regarded as an effective treatment for HCC, it is widely used for both resectable and unresectable HCC. According to the Liver Cancer Study Group of Japan [1], TAE is effective against main tumors, but not against intrahepatic metastases or portal thrombi.

Honjo et al. [11] did portal branch ligation for liver cancer in 20 patients in whom liver resection was not indicated. For the three patients who also had cirrhosis of the liver, the mean survival after portal branch ligation was 4.5 months. Histological results were not reported in their study. Laparotomy is needed for portal branch ligation. We use percutaneous transhepatic portal catheterization, which is less invasive, and have tested whether PVE before surgery has an anticancer effect.

In PVE, the catheter could be introduced up to the target portal branch with relative ease and safety. However, there were some problems concerning efficacy and safety that did not arise with TAE. Reflux of blood flow is possible in a portal branch in which there is a tumor thrombus or embolic material, because portal blood flow is slow compared with arterial blood flow. The orifice of the portal vein is larger than that of the hepatic artery. When we used either gelatin sponge or thrombin, the material shifted too readily to portal branches outside the area desired, and embolization of the branch we had planned to block was incomplete. For this reason, we chose a fibrin mixture developed as an adhesive for use in surgery, to which we added Lipiodol. We also used a balloon catheter to prevent the flow of embolic material into branches of the portal vein outside the area to be embolized. By these techniques, we could embolize the portal vein or veins we had planned to embolize completely even if the tumor thrombus was in the first branch of the portal vein. In one patient in whom the tumor thrombus was in the first branch of the portal vein, it was necessary to open the portal trunk and to close the right portal vein at the branching point during surgery, because we had to remove the embolic material from the bifurcation of the portal vein. We sometimes found that the anterior and posterior branches of the portal vein branched independently from the portal trunk. In such patients, we had to embolize these branches separately.

Immediately after PVE, portal pressure increased. In a few of the patients in whom the right portal vein was embolized, the portal pressure increased by more than 30 cm H_2O just after PVE, and their postoperative course was unsatisfactory. Therefore, PVE could be thought of as a preoperative tolerance test; if the portal pressure just after PVE is more than 30 cm H_2O, the amount of liver that is to be resected should probably be limited or some treatment other than resection should be selected. There were increases in leukocytes and slight rises in AST and ALT levels, which returned to pre-PVE levels within 2 weeks. Usually TAE was done 2 weeks before PVE and recanalization of the hepatic artery occurred within 2 weeks of TAE. In four patients in whom recanalization of the artery did not occur, there were scattered foci of infarction.

PVE causes regeneration in the embolized area of the liver and atrophy in the nonembolized area, which means that PVE decreases the resection rate. We also found that PVE allowed liver regeneration to take place in two stages, which could mean that PVE decreases overload at the early stage of liver regeneration after liver resection. Changes in some liver function tests were smaller in the patients with TAE and PVE than in patients without PVE. Therefore, PVE extends the surgical indications for patients with HCC and could make surgery safer for patients with cirrhosis of the liver.

The rate of complete necrosis of the main tumor in group AP was higher than that in the other groups. Anticancer effects for intrahepatic metastases and portal thrombi in group AP were also stronger than those in the other groups. TAE plus PVE gave fairly satisfactory effects, but viable areas still remained in some tumors, especially in intrahepatic metastases and portal thrombi, which means that surgery or other additional therapy is needed to treat the HCC. It is generally accepted that dissemination by the portal vein is one main route in the spread of HCC [12]. Theoretically, if the portal branch that might allow cancer cells to migrate is completely blocked, such metastases that arise through the portal vein should be prevented. Matsumata et al. [12] emphasized that it is important to establish a technique that prevents dissemination of cancer cells during operative manipulation. In our advanced cases in which there was a tumor thrombus in the first branch of the portal vein, only the patients in group AP survived for a long time. This means that PVE may prevent spread in such cases, especially during surgery. Thus, PVE seems to be useful not only as a preoperative treatment, but also as one medical treatment for unresectable HCC.

Acknowledgement. This study was supported in part by a Grant-in-Aid for Cancer Research from the Ministry of Health and Welfare, Japan

References

1. Liver Cancer Study Group of Japan (1990) Primary liver cancer in Japan. Clinicopathological features and results of surgical treatment. Ann Surg 211: 277–287
2. Nakashima T, Okuda K, Kojiro M, Jimi A, Yamaguchi R, Sakamoto K, Ikari T (1983) Pathology of hepatocellular carcinoma in Japan: 232 consecutive cases autopsied in ten years. Cancer 51: 863–877
3. Hsu H-C, Wu T-T, Wu M-Z, Sheu J-C, Lee C-S, Chen D-S (1988) Tumor invasiveness and prognosis in resected hepatocellular carcinoma: clinical and pathogenetic implications. Cancer 61: 2095–2099
4. Yamanaka N, Okamoto E, Toyosaka A, Mitunobu M, Fujihara S, Kato T, Fujimoto J, Oriyama T, Furukawa K, Kawamura E (1990) Prognostic factors after hepatectomy for hepatocellular carcinoma: a univariate and multivariate analysis. Cancer 65: 1104–1110
5. Hasegawa H (1983) Recent progress and results of a group study of hepatectomy following the transcatheter arterial embolization using gelatin sponge particles of CO_2 microbubbles (in Japanese). Naika 52: 555–559

6. Kinoshita H, Hirohashi K, Kubo S (1992) Preoperative portal vein embolization for hepatocellular carcinoma. In: Tobe T, Kameda H, Okudaira M, Ohto M, Endo Y, Mito M, Okamoto E, Tanikawa K, Kojiro M (eds) Primary liver cancer in Japan. Springer, Berlin Heidelberg New York pp 283–290
7. Kinoshita H, Sakai K, Hirohashi K, Igawa S, Yamasaki O, Kubo S (1986) Preoperative portal vein embolization for hepatocellular carcinoma. World J Surg 10: 803–808
8. Yamada R, Sato M, Kawabata M, Nakatsuka H, Nakamura K, Takashima S (1983) Hepatic artery embolization in 120 patients with unresectable hepatoma. Radiology 148: 397–401
9. Kinoshita H, Sakai K, Iwasa R, Hirohashi K, Kubo S, Fujio N, Lee KC (1988) Results of preoperative portal vein embolization for hepatocellular carcinoma. Osaka City Med J 34: 115–122
10. Spiessl B, Beahrs OH, Hermanek P, Hutter RVP, Scheibe O, Sobin LH, Wagner G (eds) (1990) TNM atlas. Illustrated guide to the TNM/pTNM classification of malignant tumors. Springer, Berlin Heidelberg New York, pp 98–103
11. Honjo I, Suzuki T, Ozawa K, Takasan H, Kitamura O, Ishikawa T (1975) Ligation of a branch of the portal vein for carcinoma of the liver. Am J Surg 130: 296–302
12. Matsumata T, Kanematsu T, Takenaka K, Yoshida Y, Nishizaki T, Sugimachi K (1989) Patterns of intrahepatic recurrence after curative resection of hepatocellular carcinoma. Hepatology 9: 457–460

Fibrin Sealing in Liver and Spleen Surgery

H. W. WACLAWICZEK

Abstract

For a long time the danger of diffuse bleedings after resections and traumas of liver and spleen, which were hard to control, was the reason for a reserved attitude towards indications for surgical interventions in these parenchymatous organs. As a result of the rapid development of screening diagnosis, the improvement of perioperative intensive care medicine, and the increasing refinement of operation techniques, the incidence of critical bleedings has been reduced. Fibrin sealing, by which especially diffuse parenchymatous bleedings can be treated efficiently and safely, has played an important part in liver and spleen surgery of the past 15 years [5–8].

Liver Traumas

Under certain conditions, especially in children, a primarily conservative procedure is recommended for the treatment of liver trauma. Eligible for this method are hemodynamically stable patients whose computer tomogram shows simple parenchymatous injuries or intrahepatic hematomas. About 10–20 % of all patients fulfill these criteria [6].

Approximately 90 % of penetrating and 60 % of blunt liver traumas belong to stages I and II. The therapeutic spectrum ranges from simple examination to the adaptation suture of superficial ruptures and the sealing of these injuries with fibrin glue.

In 42 cases of superficial liver traumas, we used the method of fibrin sealing for hemostasis. Following the precise ligature of larger arterial or venous vessels and bile ducts, the wound fissure was filled with fibrin sealant (1–4 ml); then the wound fissures were adapted with one to three sutures (collagen bands). Thus, efficient hemostasis could be achieved intraoperatively (Fig. 1). During the postoperative course only one case of a subcapsular hematoma occurred, which was treated conservatively. None of the patients died.

For liver traumas of stages III and IV ($n = 19$), the following procedure was chosen: In the case of destroyed hepatic tissue, liver resections including hemihepatectomies ($n = 12$) were carried out. After mostly atypical resection of the ruptured liver tissue, the ligature of large vessels or bile ducts, respec-

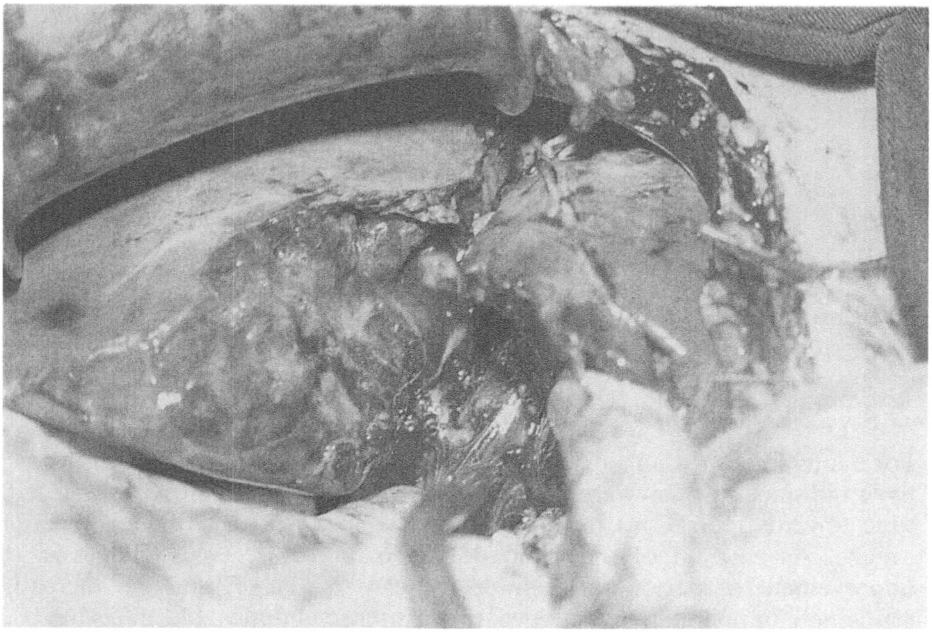

Fig. 1. Sealed liver rupture adapted by collagen bands

tively, was performed. Then the diffusely bleeding resection surface was sealed with a thick fibrin film (Fig. 2) and additionally covered with a large collagen fleece soaked in fibrin sealant.

In cases where the vena cava or big hepatic veins were ruptured, primary closure of these vessels with sutures was done ($n = 8$). In these seriously shocked and mostly polytraumatized patients, a tamponade of the upper abdomen with abdominal baths was then carried out due to heavy bleeding out of the liver tissue and/or the retroperitoneum; the abdominal wound was only closed temporarily. When the shock had stabilized, relaparotomy was performed after 1–3 days, the tamponade was removed, and the destroyed hepatic tissue resected. Finally, these resection surfaces were treated with fibrin sealant and covered with collagen fleece.

Results

Out of the group with primarily resected liver traumas, none of the patients died; in one case a biliary fistula occurred, which ceased after 1 week.

Three out of the eight patients with extensive liver traumas and large vessel injuries died postoperatively due to traumatic shock. In another case rebleeding after fibrin sealing of the liver rupture occurred; therefore, a relaparotomy was required for further sealing of the lesion.

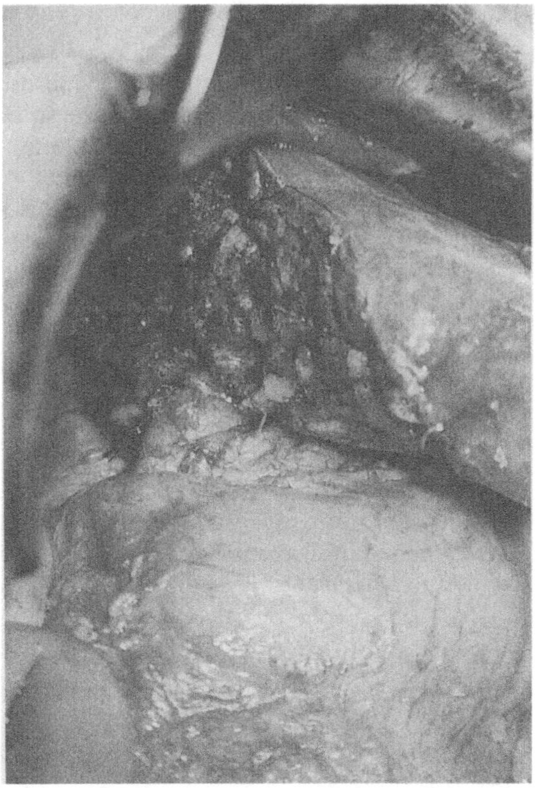

Fig. 2. Liver resection surface covered with a thick fibrin film

Liver Tumors

In 58 cases of benign ($n = 17$) or malignant ($n = 41$) tumors of the liver, resections (37 segmental, 21 hemihepatectomies) were performed. In all these cases – after mostly atypical resection of the hepatic tissue by electrocoagulation and recently also using the ultrasound knife (CUSA; Cavitron, Stanford) – the resection surface was sealed with fibrin glue (2–5 ml) and covered with a collagen fleece. Thus, exact hemostasis of even diffuse bleeding could be achieved and in addition the operation area was drained.

Results

One patient died postoperatively due to liver dystrophy as a result of an extended resection (lethality, 1.7%). Another female patient had to undergo relaparotomy because of rebleeding on the first postoperative day and the resection surface had to be sealed again with fibrin. In all the other cases, no surgical complications were observed.

Spleen Traumas

For long time splenectomy was considered the best method for treating traumatic and intraoperative injuries of the spleen. This was due to the fact that this organ was not regarded as a vital one. Animal experiments and clinical research proved, however, that splenectomy caused considerable disorder in terms of immunity resistance and this disorder supports favorable conditions for the formation of sepsis (overwhelming postsplenectomy infection, OPSI). The frequency of local complications, such as subphrenic abscesses, increases following splenectomies [1–4]. The preservation of the spleen is made possible by use of fibrin sealant.

Since 1989 we have always taken fibrin sealing into account for hemostasis, following traumas and intraoperative lesions of the spleen.

Fibrin sealing was used in 98 cases of traumatic and 22 cases of intraoperative lesions of the spleen. In most of these cases ($n = 114$), the fibrin sealant was applied directly into the wound fissure. After about 5 min of digital compression, the ruptured organ was plugged by application of a collagen fleece soaked in fibrin sealant (Fig. 3). In six additional cases, a partial splenectomy was performed by sealing the resection surface with fibrin glue.

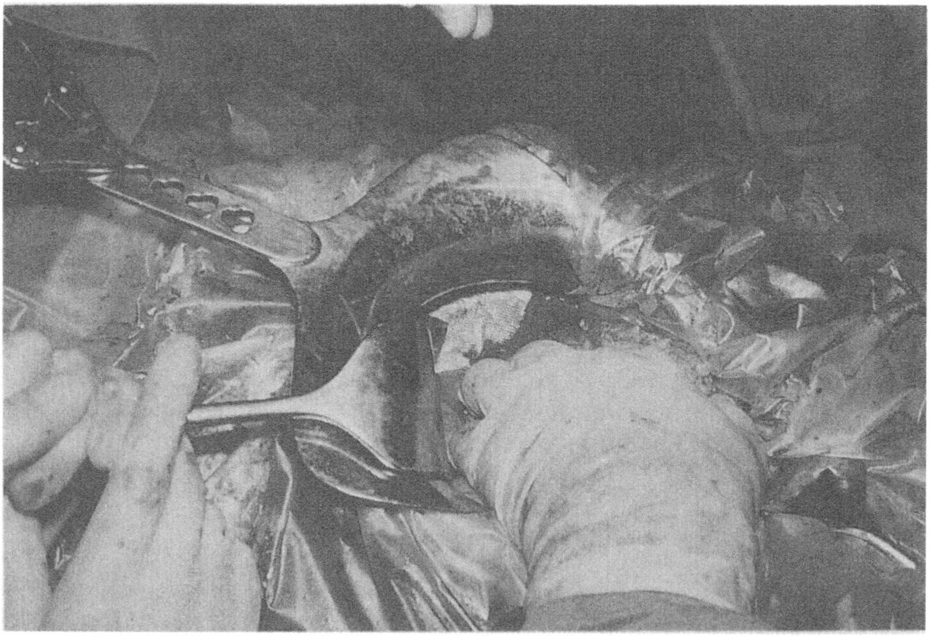

Fig. 3. Spleen injury plugged by a collagen fleece soaked in fibrin sealant

Results

In eight cases, either intraoperatively ($n = 6$) or postoperatively ($n = 2$) a removal of the glued spleen due to the extended ruptures had to be carried out, but in more than 90% of cases, the organ was preserved. Apart from a subphrenic abscess, which was drained by transcutaneous puncture, no further postoperative complications occurred in the other patients.

Discussion

Adequate use of conventional surgical techniques with ligatures and sutures is the major requirement for the control of hemorrhage and biliary leakage following hepatic and splenic traumas and after partial liver resections. However, in a significant number of cases, arterial oozing hemorrhage and bile fistulas persist, thus increasing postoperative complication rates. Any further aggressive attempt to complete hemostasis, such as the use of deep ligature by thick, nonabsorbable strands, compresses additional vessels and leads to large tissue compartments that are hypoperfused and, consequently, damaged by necrosis.

In the past, different adjuvant methods for the control of hemorrhage have been developed. However, definitive superiority of one of these methods has yet to be proved.

Therefore, the use of fibrin sealant is a feasible and safe method in the control of bleeding in liver and spleen surgery. If a surgeon is familiar with this technique, particularly with details of application modalities, the success rate should exceed 90% for traumatic injuries, as shown by our results.

The technique of preliminary vascular ligation and covering the injury or resection surface with fibrin sealant in combination with a collagen fleece has proven very reliable and safe in our experience. It avoids tissue damage as well as any postoperative oozing. Nevertheless, our low complication rate illustrates that this requires a reliable surgical method [7, 8].

References

1. Leonhard AS, Giebink GS, Baesel TJ, Krivit W (1980) The overwhelming postsplenectomy sepsis problem. World J Surg 4: 423
2. Mitterstieler G, Müller W, Hammerer I, Höpfel-Kreiner I (1978) Disseminierte intravasale Gerinnung bei Pneumokokkensepsis nach Splenektomie. Z Kinderchir 25: 8
3. Pimpl W, Wayand W (1983) Ergebnisse der experimentellen Autotransplantation von Milzgewebe beim Hausschwein. Acta Chir Austriaca 15: 1
4. Scheele J (1981) Erste klinische Erfahrungen mit der Fibrinklebung bei traumatischer und intraoperativer Milzverletzung. Chirurg 52: 531
5. Scheele J (1986) Splenic salvage by the use of fibrin tissue adhesive. In: Schlag G, Redl H (eds) General surgery and abdominal surgery. Springer, Berlin Heidelberg New York, pp 96–108
6. Scheele J, Gall FP (1992) Blutstillungstechniken an Milz und Leber – Stellenwert im therapeutischen Gesamtkonzept. Jahrbuch der Chirurgie, Biermann, pp 219–240

7. Waclawiczek HW, Boeckl O (1986) Clinical experience with fibrin sealing in general and thoracic surgery. In: Schlag G, Redl H (eds) General surgery and abdominal surgery. Springer, Berlin Heidelberg New York, pp 63–71
8. Waclawiczek HW, Meiser G (1990) La colle de fibrine en chirurgie. Lyon Chir 86 (5): 412–419

Indications and Techniques for Fibrin Sealing in Spleen Surgery

S. Uranüs

Abstract

Surgical treatment of splenic lesions aims to save the organ in order to preserve hematological and immunological functions. The choice of surgical procedure will depend on the type and degree of injury in trauma cases and on the respective disease in elective cases. Any number of surgical treatment options for the various situations are available. During a period of 56 months, we administered organ-conserving treatment to 69 adults for a variety of indications. Four trauma patients were managed nonoperatively and 65 underwent surgery. Coagulation was used in three trauma cases with first- and second-degree ruptures. For the remaining patients, fibrin sealing was the main treatment or an adjuvant along with other surgical procedures. Fibrin sealing alone was used in 19 cases. In 28 cases, we used mesh splenorrhaphy for severe bursting ruptures and stapler resection was used in 15 further cases. Primary hemostasis was achieved in all the trauma patients. There was only one case in which a second operation was required for postoperative bleeding and there was one further case that required a secondary splenectomy. Blood transfusions were never required in elective cases, and none of them required further surgery. Postoperative laboratory work and scintigraphy showed optimal splenic perfusion and preservation of hematological and immunological function in all patients. Thus, we can say that spleen preservation using fibrin glue as monotherapy or adjuvant to other techniques can be safely performed in adult patients, either after a variety of injuries or in elective cases. The risk of postoperative bleeding is 1.5 %, which is less than for splenectomy. For safe performance of spleen-preserving surgery, the spleen must be fully mobilized and visualized during surgery.

Introduction

The spleen is one of the few organs whose morphology and function long remained unstudied and whose real importance went unrecognized. In antiquity, the spleen was thought to belong to the digestive tract; this view persisted into the seventeenth century. It was not until 1686 that Malpighi demonstrated the follicular and trabecular structure of the spleen and the fact that it had its own arterial and venous circulation (cited in [12]). In 1919, Morris and Bullock first showed the influence of the spleen in resistance to infection and found an increased mortality in splenectomized rats inoculated with the rat plague bacillus [9] O'Donnel reported the first human case of fatal postsplenectomy sepsis in 1929 [11]. In 1952, King and Shumacker concluded that removal of the spleen for spherocytosis in five infants aged less than 1 year led to severe infections [6].

The first splenectomy was performed in Palermo in 1549 by Zaccarello of Palo (cited in [8]). However, due to the unsatisfactory course of splenectomies before the turn of the present century, mortality with clinically recognized splenic injuries was nearly 100 %. With the introduction of asepsis in surgery and standardization of the surgical technique in the 1930s, mortality decreased to 27 %. Thus, splenectomy became the gold standard treatment for splenic injury [1]. The real revolution in surgical handling was introduced by the pioneering work of Leon Morgenstern and the Brazilian surgeon Marcel Campos Christo in the early 1960s and 1970s. Christo first reported experimental segmental splenectomy in animals. Then he applied these techniques to eight patients with splenic injuries [2]. In 1966, Morgenstern reported subtotal splenectomy in myelofibrosis [7]. These publications on partial splenic conservation in trauma and massive splenomegaly attracted the attention not only of pediatric, but also of general surgeons. Morgenstern's work especially has had a significant impact on acceptance of splenic preservation. Since the mid-1970s, the routine splenectomy procedure has gradually changed, and today conservation of the organ can be seen as an established method. Treatment options now range from nonoperative treatment to splenorrhaphy and hemisplenectomy [16].

Tissue sealing presents a valuable alternative. Of the adhesives currently available, the most suitable for treating splenic lesions is fibrin glue. A major advantage of the adhesive procedure is that it can be combined with all other techniques as an additional hemostatic measure.

Patients and Methods

Between May 1, 1987 and December 31, 1991, 69 adults underwent organ-conserving splenic surgery (Table 1). Fibrin adhesives were used either alone or with other measures in all patients with the exception of seven traumas, including four nonoperatively managed cases and three treated with coagulation. Among the 62 patients treated with fibrin glue, 19 had first- and second-degree splenic injuries (seven traumatic and 12 accidental ruptures); here, the sealing technique was used alone. It was used supplementally in the remaining 28 mesh splenorrhaphy and 15 stapler resection patients. Fibrin glue was thus applied in 62 cases or 90 % of the 69 spleen-preserving operations.

Table 1. Spleen-preserving operations

Diagnosis	Patients (*n*)	Patients (%)	Non-operative conservative	Operative: Adhesives	Operative: Coagulation	Operative: Mesh	Operative: Stapler
Traumatic rupture	46	67	4	7	2	28	5
Accidental rupture	16	23	–	12	1	–	3
Therapeutic resection	5	7	–	–	–	–	5
Diagnostic resection	2	3	–	–	–	–	2
Total	69	100	4 (6%)	19 (28%)	3 (4%)	28 (40%)	15 (22%)

1.5.1987–31.12.1991, Department of Surgery, University of Graz.

Fibrin Glue

Fibrin glue as monotherapy is used preferentially in the treatment of first- and second-degree splenic ruptures. The bleeding parenchymal surface is first tamponed briefly with a warm towel; then fibrin is applied and, when necessary, collagen fleece can be pressed upon it for a few minutes. Compressing the parenchymal surface before the adhesive procedure serves to free the surface of blood while the fibrin is being applied. This can be supplemented by brief and careful digital compression of the hilus. When the blood flow is too heavy, both of these measures – digital compression of the hilus and parenchymal tamponade – should be performed, otherwise the adhesive and/or the collagen fleece will not stick. Here it has proved advantageous to use a compressed-air device (Tissomat, Immuno, Vienna). First, air alone is sprayed before the fibrin is applied. This creates a surface that is free of blood and nearly dry (Fig. 1). Alternatively the adhesive components can be applied sequentially to the collagen fleece. The hemostyptic must, however, be compressed locally for a few minutes. This keeps the area free of blood during the polymerization phase of the adhesive, preventing the hemostyptic from being washed away and ensuring that a hematoma does not develop underneath.

Mesh Splenorrhaphy

We used this technique to treat third-degree bursting ruptures. They are usually deep lacerations not only on the convex, but also on the concave surface. They sometimes extend to the hilus and cause severe bleeding. An important prerequisite in this technique as well is the full mobilization of the injured spleen and its rotation into the abdominal incision. A piece of compressive mesh (Vicryl, Ethicon; 28 × 18 cm, gauge 0.5 mm) is applied to form an impression of the injured spleen. Then, an absorbable 0-gauge thread (Vicryl, Ethicon) is

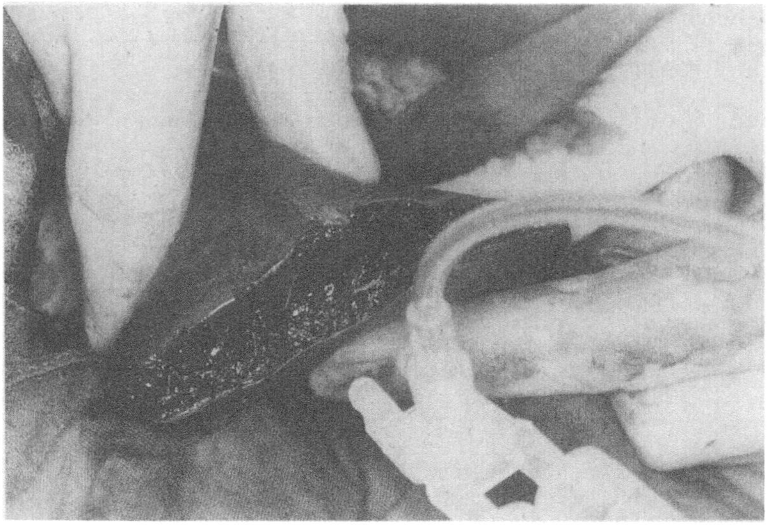

Fig. 1. Fibrin sealing with the Tissomat sprayer on the resected edge after hemisplenectomy

drawn through the mesh to form a pouch of appropriate size. The spleen is inserted into the pouch and the thread is pulled together and knotted so that the pressure of the mesh is uniform over the entire surface of the organ. It is extremely important that the pouch be slightly smaller than the spleen itself, so that the thread lies on the acute and obtuse margin when it has been pulled taut. Because of the tension of the mesh on the hilar aspect, the splenic tissue forms a cone over the hilus. The mesh does not touch the tissue on the visceral aspect and so there is a sufficiently large space around the hilus for vessels to enter and emerge; even the smallest vessels are not constricted. The conization itself compresses the splenic parenchyma on the concave surface, facilitating the desired hemostasis even in deep ruptures of this surface. On the convex diaphragmatic surface, the mesh lies taut over the surface and compresses the ruptured parenchyma. By compressing the parenchyma from the outside, hemostasis is achieved without affecting circulation within the organ. Any slight oozing of blood through the holes in the mesh will be arrested with fibrin glue applied with the Tissomat sprayer as described above (Fig. 2).

Before the spleen is replaced in its fossa, the ligaments are carefully inspected and any bleeding stopped. The spleen is fixed in its fossa with two or three single sutures on the diaphragm and the retroperitoneal connective tissue to prevent torsion. The splenic fossa is not usually drained, except in cases where the opening of hollow organs contaminates the abdominal cavity.

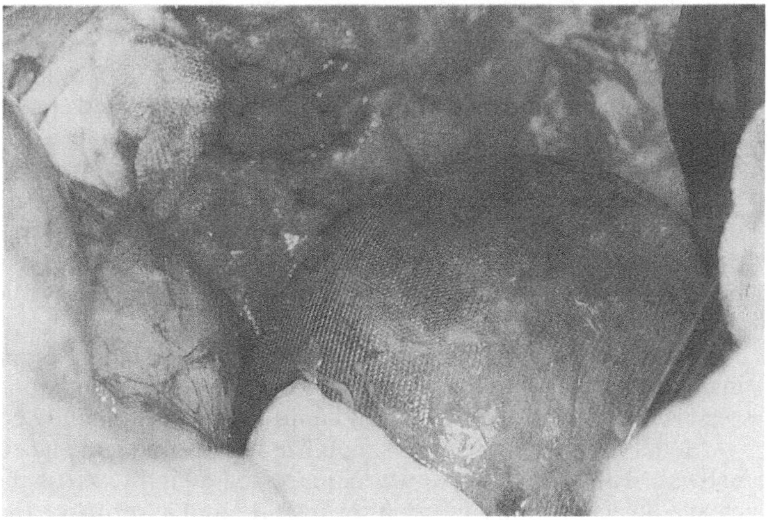

Fig. 2. Polyglactin-910 mesh after successful splenorrhaphy and application of fibrin glue

Stapler Resection

In 15 cases the stapler was used for partial resection. There were five grade II and III traumatic ruptures (Table 2). The lesions were limited to one pole or to half of the spleen. Three patients with iatrogenic injuries underwent lower-pole

Table 2. Treatment of Traumatic Splenic Rupture

Surgical Method	(*n*)	%	Degree of injury 0	I	II	III	IV
Conservative	4	(6)	4	–	–	–	–
Fibrin glue	7	(11)	–	5	2	–	–
Coagulation	2	(3)	–	–	2	–	–
Mesh-Splenorrhaphy	28	(45)	–	–	4	24	–
Stapler-Resection	5	(8)	–	–	5	–	–
Primary Splenectomy	17	(27)	–	–	–	–	17
[Secondary Splenectomy	2	(3)	–	–	–	2	–]
Total	63		4 (6%)	5 (8%)	13 (20%)	24 (40%)	17 (26%)

1. 5. 1987–31. 12. 1991, Department of Surgery, University of Graz.

resection. In five cases, we performed a therapeutic resection for isolated splenic cysts. The cysts included a mesothelial cyst, an epidermoid cyst, an intralienal pancreas cyst, and two post traumatic pseudocysts. Two patients had a diagnostic partial resection, and both showed isolated splenomegaly. Hematological studies and marrow puncture could not confirm the diagnosis of a hematological disorder.

In all cases of elective surgery, prior to mobilization of the spleen the bursa omentalis was opened via the ligamentum gastrocolicum, followed by prehilar presentation and snaring of the splenic artery. Blood supply was temporarily interrupted during the resection by a tourniquet, which was released as soon as the staples had been applied.

In the trauma cases, we left out the time-consuming procedure of preparing and snaring the splenic artery. In these cases, the surgeon compressed the vessels digitally on the hilus until hemostasis had ultimately been achieved.

In all cases, the spleen was mobilized all around and placed on the abdominal wall. The splenic tissue was compressed digitally across the normal parenchyma adjacent to the injury after ligature and severing of the respective vessels (Fig. 3). That pushed the parenchyma toward the damaged segment that would later be removed. Only two lobes of the capsule and vascular cords of connective tissue remained between the surgeon's fingers. This was where the stapler and the staples were applied (Fig. 4). In trauma cases, the extent of the resection is determined by the injury.

The cystic lesions were opened before resection and the contents suctioned off after removal of a sample. This served to prevent accidental contamination of the abdominal cavity. The cysts are generally removed by blunt dissection with the finger-fracture technique (Fig. 5). Care is taken to remove all

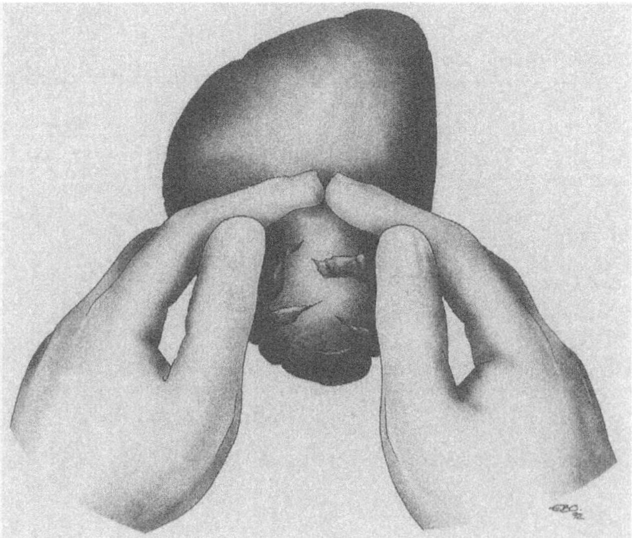

Fig. 3. Digital compression of the normal parenchyma adjacent to the injured part of the spleen

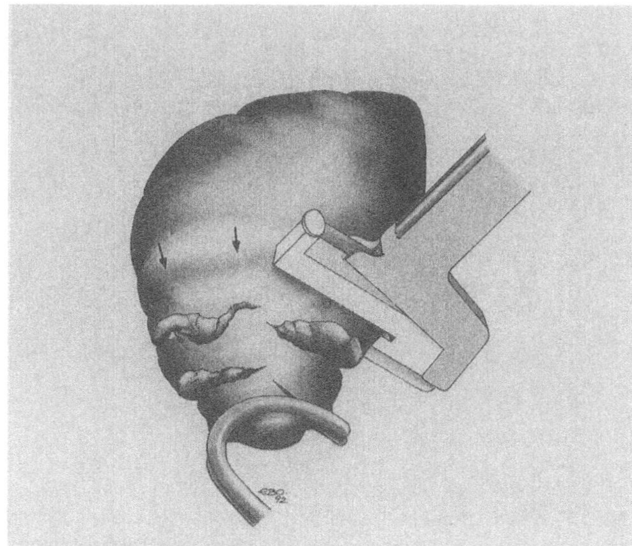

Fig. 4. Positioning of the stapler on the compression line *(arrows)*

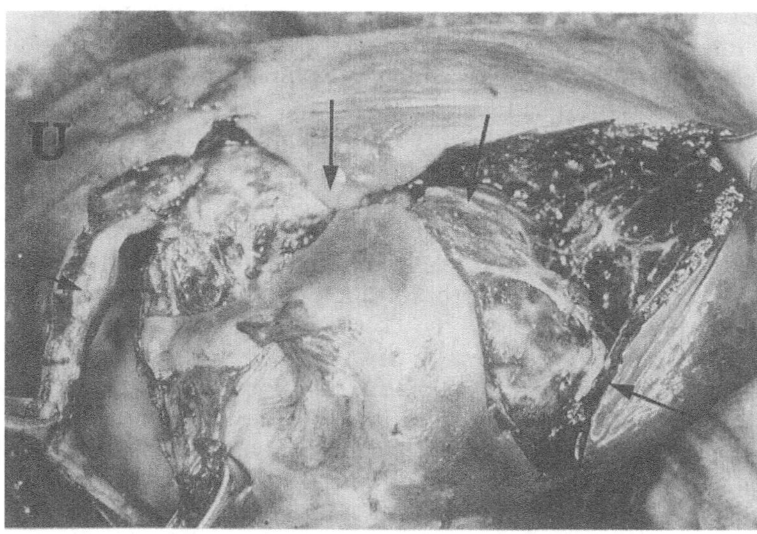

Fig. 5. Large congenital cyst in the middle segment of the spleen (arrows). *U* upper pole

remnants of cystic epithelium. Then the tourniquet is loosened and the spurting vessels are tied off. Only then are the stapler and the staples applied (Fig. 6). Theoretically, the cysts do not have to be opened before resection. This can, however, pose problems with congenital cysts as they may have processes reaching into the neighboring parenchyma that are not outwardly apparent. If these processes are not completely removed in the course of a

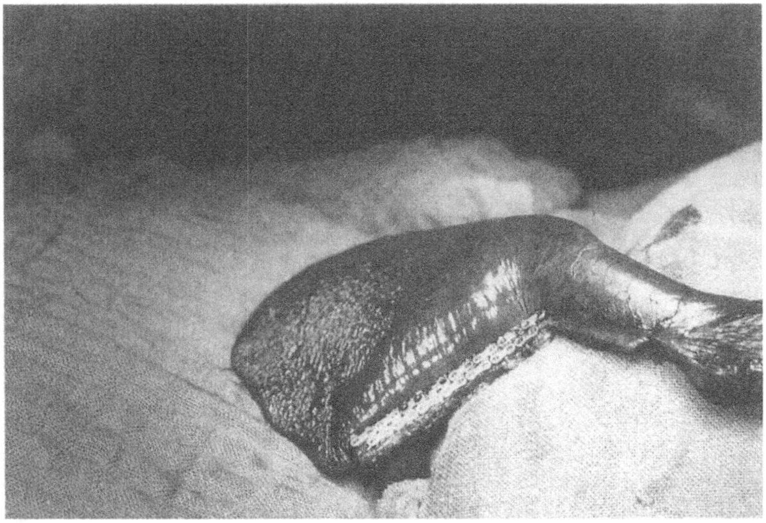

Fig. 6. Upper pole after removal of the cyst. Double row of absorbable staples on the resected edge

closed resection, there may be a recurrence. On the other hand, if the resection is too generous, too much functional tissue will be lost. We have found that open cystectomy with subsequent adaptation of the parenchymal edges using the stapler is most suitable.

In all cases, fibrin glue (Tissucol, Immuno, Vienna, Austria) was applied to the resected edges with a compressed-air sprayer (Tissomat, Immuno, Vienna, Austria) and tamponed with collagen fleece.

We used the TA-55 stapler (Auto Suture Instruments, Norwalk, CN, USA) 14 times and the TA-90 stapler once. Depending on the thickness of the tissue, we twice used 3.5 nonresorbable stapler units (height of closed staple 1.5 mm), and in the other 13 cases, the Polysorb 55 disposable unit (United States Surgical Corporation, Norwalk, CN, USA) with absorbable staples. In three cases, these were No. 170 staples with a height of 4.3 mm when closed. In the remaining resections, we used No. 200 staples with a height of 5 mm when closed. The choice of staple unit always depended on the thickness of the splenic parenchyma. To save as much of the organ as possible, we make a V-shaped resection with the TA-55. Only in one case of cyst resection was it more advantageous to make a straight cut, so we used the TA-90.

Results

In all cases, primarily satisfactory hemostasis on the injured site or on the resected edge was achieved. Fibrin glue was effective in achieving hemostasis on the first application in all 12 accidental injuries. In four of seven traumatic ruptures we also used collagen fleece as an additional hemostatic agent.

Two patients in the group of 28 mesh splenorrhaphy cases died of their other multiple injuries 4 h and 5 days, respectively, after successful spleen preservation. In two other cases, the spleen was removed secondarily 8 h and 7 days, respectively, after primary conservation. In the first case, the patient also had, in addition to his third-degree splenic rupture, multiple fractures of the extremities, bilateral thoracic contusion, ruptured liver, pancreatic hematoma, and lacerations of the terminal mesenteric and transverse mesocolon. An emergency laparotomy was performed and the abdominal injuries were treated without resection of the colon. The spleen was conserved with mesh splenorrhaphy. The injured extremities were stabilized 24 h later. Later, the patient developed multiorgan failure and persistent ileus. CT scans of the thorax and abdomen failed to clarify the situation. The patient's condition was too poor to permit splenic scintigraphy to exclude a total splenic necrosis due to excessive compression by the mesh. On the seventh day after spleen preservation, a second laparotomy was performed. The spleen in its compressive mesh was covered with a thin layer of fibrin that adhered firmly to it and so it was not possible to assess with certainty the viability of the underlying organ. We thus decided to perform a splenectomy, as there was no safe way to determine the viability of the organ. Histology showed narrow necrotic strips along the old ruptures, but not the total necrosis we had feared. The patient improved with further intensive care and was finally discharged in satisfactory condition after 6 weeks. With the advantage of hindsight, we can say that splenectomy would not have been necessary in this case. It was, however, a valuable experience at the time when we began our work with mesh splenorrhaphy.

In the second of these two cases, a repeat laparotomy was required 8 h after the first operation, due to bleeding. An incompletely mobilized spleen was found; the mesh pouch had slipped off and lay next to the organ. The surgeon who had performed the initial operation was inexperienced in the techniques of reparative splenic surgery and had failed to completely mobilize the organ; a splenectomy was then required.

In all 15 cases with stapler resection of the spleen, satisfactory hemostasis of the resected edge was achieved. The slight oozing of blood from between the staples could always be arrested, and a second laparotomy was never required. The splenic surgery lasted an average of 20 min. Blood transfusion was not required in any of the seven elective partial resections. With the traumatic and accidental ruptures where stapler resection was performed, we cannot say anything objective about the amount of blood transfused, as these cases also involved other injuries and/or organs. Both the trauma patients and those with accidental ruptures whose spleens were conserved surgically showed no significant difference in the amount of blood transfused as compared to splenectomy patients.

The repeat – laparotomy rate was 3 % (two of 65 patients) and the postoperative bleeding rate was 1.5 % (one of 65 patients). We did not lose any patients to surgical complications. It is difficult to give any precise data about blood loss from these organ-conserving procedures due to the overall complexity of these multiple-trauma cases. In general, we saw no significant difference in the amount of blood transfused as compared to multiple-trauma cases with splenectomy.

All patients subjected to orthotopic spleen conservation underwent laboratory tests and scintigraphy 4 weeks and 6 months postoperatively. Laboratory tests included differential blood count, immune globulins, complement component C3, and interleukin-2. These tests were always within normal limits both upon discharge and upon follow-up after 6 months. Splenic scintigraphy with heat-damaged autologous erythrocytes marked with Tc-99m always showed good function, with small activity deficits corresponding to the degree of trauma.

Discussion

The spleen is the largest lymphatic organ and it has only efferent lymph vessels, which originate in the white pulp. The spleen is directly connected to the blood circulatory system. These are the features that make it so important in the defence against hematogenic infections. Optimal results in retaining organ function are only obtained when a sufficiently large spleen (at least 25 % of the initial size) is conserved orthotopically.

Organ-conserving surgery on the spleen seeks to retain the important functions of this organ in the immune system, but it should not be done at any price. In multiple-trauma cases especially, the organ-conserving operation should not take much longer than a splenectomy would, and the technique used should not require excessive blood transfusion. The basic prerequisites for fast and uncomplicated conservation of the spleen are a good view with generous exposure of the surgical field and complete mobilization of the organ. Only when these requirements have been met can one of the techniques available today be applied. The choice of procedure depends not only on the clinical findings, but also on the case history, the surgeon's experience in splenic surgery, and the equipment available at the respective hospital.

Fibrin glue is effective either as a primary agent or as an adjuvant for obtaining hemostasis. No complications resulted from glue itself, although hepatitis and acquired immunodeficiency syndrome (AIDS) remain potential long-term problems. This risk is no greater than that of a single-unit blood transfusion [10]. We suggest that fibrin glue is an effective adjunct for hemostasis either in trauma or in elective spleen surgery.

Orthotopic conservation of first- and second-degree splenic injuries can usually be accomplished without difficulty with the various suture, sealing, and coagulation techniques, but these often do not suffice for third-degree trauma. Third-degree injuries feature deep tears extending to the segmental arteries on both the hilar and diaphragmatic surfaces. Local hemostatic measures are not very useful for these bursting ruptures. Sutures, coagulation, and application of adhesives are too time-consuming and often do not achieve the desired hemostasis. Upon admission, patients with severe bursting ruptures generally have other injuries, have lost a lot of blood, and are usually in shock; thus, reconstruction and conservation of the organ should not take much more time than would a splenectomy.

Until Delany's publication in 1982, the use of the various heterologous tissue substitutes in abdominal surgery was limited to the covering of defects

[3, 5]. Delany was first to use a resorbable synthetic mesh to repair splenic ruptures in experimental animals, fixing the mesh to the splenic parenchyma with a series of running and single button stitches [3]. In the six clinical cases he reported in 1985, the mesh was sometimes even fastened with stitches going all the way through the parenchyma [4].

Tribble et al. published another version of mesh splenorrhaphy in 1987 [13]. With this technique, the mesh was slit to the middle; the hilar vessels were pulled through this slit, which was enlarged to a circle in the center of the mesh. The mesh was then sewed together with a running stitch on the convex surface [13]. We found that Delany's sutures passing through the parenchyma can lead to new tears and bleeding. A mesh pulled together on the convex surface of the spleen (Tribble's method) and stretched tight to compress the tissue will also compress the hilar and segmental vessels on the hilar surface. Otherwise, the compression is insufficient and there will be further bleeding. The basic idea here was good, but the technique needed improvement. First in experimental work and then in clinical practice, we were able to show that this method produces satisfactory hemostasis in severe third-degree splenic ruptures [14, 15]. The operation is simple and quickly performed. The possibility of combining this method with the adhesive procedure enhances its reliability.

A partial resection of the spleen may be necessary with second- and third-degree ruptures limited to one pole, benign cysts, and pathological processes that have spread to the spleen from neighboring organs (e.g., intralienal pancreatic pseudocyst). Resection with a stapler is an addition to the program of organ preservation. It represents a valuable alternative to the sutured partial splenectomy or splenorrhaphy [17]. The greatest advantages of this technique are the simplicity of use, the practicality of the instrument itself, and the reduction in time and blood transfusions required for surgery.

References

1. Beal SL, Spisso JM (1988) The risk of splenorrhaphy. Arch Surg 123: 1158
2. Christo MC (1962) Segmental resection of the spleen: report on the first eight cases operated on. O Hospital (Rio) 62: 575
3. Delany HM (1982) Splenic capping: an experimental study of a new technique for splenorrhaphy using woven polyglycolic acid mesh. Ann Surg 196: 187
4. Delany HM, Rudavsky AZ, Lan S (1985) Preliminary clinical experience with the use of absorbable mesh splenorrhaphy. J Trauma 25: 909
5. Eigler FW, Gross E, Klaes W (1985) Resorbierbare Kunststoffnetze in der Abdominalchirurgie. Chirurg 56: 376
6. King H, Shumacker HB (1952) Splenic studies. Ann Surg 136: 239
7. Morgenstern L (1966) Subtotal splenectomy in myelofibrosis. Surg 60: 336
8. Morgenstern L (1986) Evolution of splenic surgery: from mythology to modernity. Contemporary Surgery 29: 15
9. Morris DH, Bullock FD (1919) The importance of the spleen in resistance to infection. Ann Surg 76: 513
10. Ochsner MG, Maniscaleo-Theberge ME, Champion HR (1990) Fibrin glue as a hemostatic agent in hepatic and splenic trauma. J Trauma 30: 884
11. O'Donnel JF (1929) The value of splenectomy in Banti's Disease. Br Med J 1: 854

12. Schreiber HW, Schumpelick V (1976) Zur Geschichte der Milz-Chirurgie. Med Welt 27: 1212
13. Tribble CG, Joob AW, Barone GW, Rodgers BM (1987) A new technique for wrapping the injured spleen with polyglactin mesh. The American Surgeon 53: 663
14. Uranüs S, Kronberger L, Beham A, Neumayer K, Kröll W, Aktuna D (1990) Neue organerhaltende Techniken beim drittgradigen Milztrauma. Eine experimentelle Studie. Z Exp Chir Transplant künstl Organe 23: 7
15. Uranüs S, Kronberger L, Pinter H, Stenzl W (1990) Klinischer Einsatz neuer organerhaltender Techniken in der Milzchirurgie. Chirurg 61: 116
16. Uranüs S (1994) The spleen and its current surgery. Zuckschwerdt, Munich
17. Uranüs S, Kronberger L (1994) Partial splenic resection using the TA-Stapler. Am J Surg (in press)

Fibrin Sealing for Intrahepatic Hepaticojejunostomy – A New Technical Modification

P. Moeschl, D. Oturandlar, and A. Kroiss

Abstract

Resection of the hepatic bifurcation for Klatskin tumors necessarily requires intrahepatic anastomosis. Although these tumors grow slowly, the average resectability rate is only about 20%. This situation may well be due to major technical problems concerning resection and reconstruction.

Although various methods have been described, reconstruction of the bile flow is still a major problem. Mucosa-to-mucosa anastomosis with resorbable monofilament material, mucosal flap technique supported by positioning sutures to the liver capsule, and omentum flap technique with long-term intraluminal stenting and a combined extracorporeal and inner drainage have been tried. Moreover, "unnecessary" liver resections of the right, left, or quadrate lobe performed only for technical reasons are used for a better exposure of the hepatic ducts during the anastomosing procedure. Nevertheless, all these techniques are still problematic if the resection margin has to be positioned up against the secondary and tertiary hepatic convergences. This situation is reflected by a high complication rate, especially late complications such as infection and stenosis. The stenosis rate is still about 20%.

In our search for a better solution, we tried fibrin sealing for hepaticojejunostomy. In a case of type III tumor (Bismuth), we had to resect up to the tertiary convergences. Transhepatic intraluminal balloon catheters were used for approximation of a Roux-en-Y loop intrahepatically. The catheters also functioned as short-term stenting with inner and extracorporeal bile drainage. Fibrin sealing was used to perform a close anastomosis as well as to fix the bowel loop within the liver.

The postoperative outcome was totally unproblematic. As early as 2½ weeks after the operation, the balloon catheters could be removed and the patient was discharged. One year follow-up of the patient showed a well-functioning anastomosis by bile X-ray, Tc-99, HIDA scan and liver function tests.

We therefore recommend fibrin sealing for this indication as a further step to improve liver surgery.

Introduction

Because of their localization, cancers of the hepatic bifurcation, so-called Klatskin tumors [12], are still a technical problem for surgery. This is reflected by a radical resection rate of only about 20 % or less [5, 22] as well as a high mortality rate. Although the operative mortality of approximately 40 % in earlier reports [1, 9, 14, 18] has markedly declined, it still reaches 17 % or more even in bigger series at specialized centers [5, 13]. Inadequate access to the intrahepatic ducts and the difficulty in anastomosing the secondary and tertiary convergencies of the hepatic ducts with a jejunal loop still seem to be the major technical problems. Therefore, biliary fistulas, cholangitis, sepsis, and septicemia are the most frequent early complications [2, 14, 15, 18], and restenoses in 10 %–30 % of cases and chronic cholangitis are the most important late problems [16, 17, 21]. Up to now, a lot of technical variations and modifications have been tried in an attempt to solve the problems of a deep intrahepatic hepaticojejunostomy. They will be discussed following the detailed description of our technical modification, which uses and combines the experiences of these earlier techniques.

Material and Methods

A type III Klatskin tumor as described by Bismuth [2], which extended to both hepatic ducts, had to be operated in a 72-year-old lady (Fig. 1). The tumor, a well-differentiated adenocarcinoma at the stage T1b, was removed by a RO

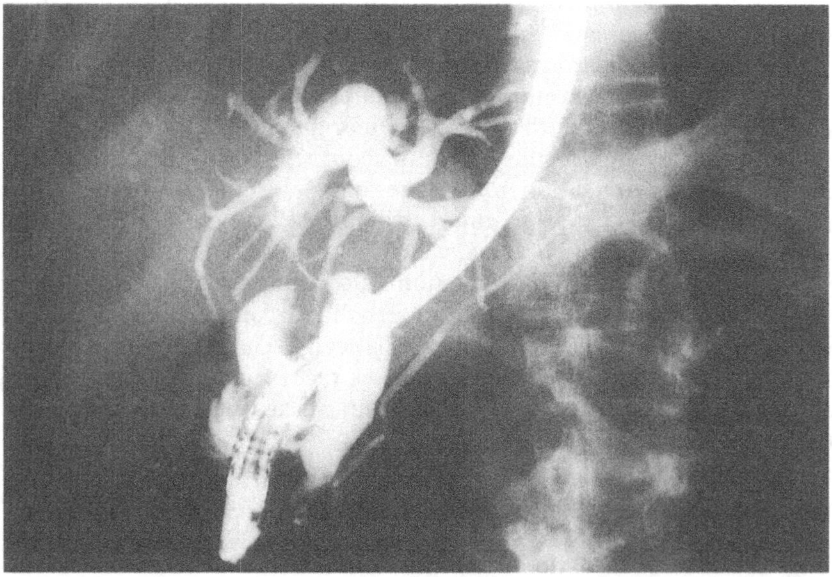

Fig. 1. Type III Klatskin tumor in a 72-year-old patient, totally occluding the bile flow. The hepatic ducts are filled with contrast medium by percutaneous puncture previously. The choledochus is shown by endoscopic retrograde cholangiopancreatography

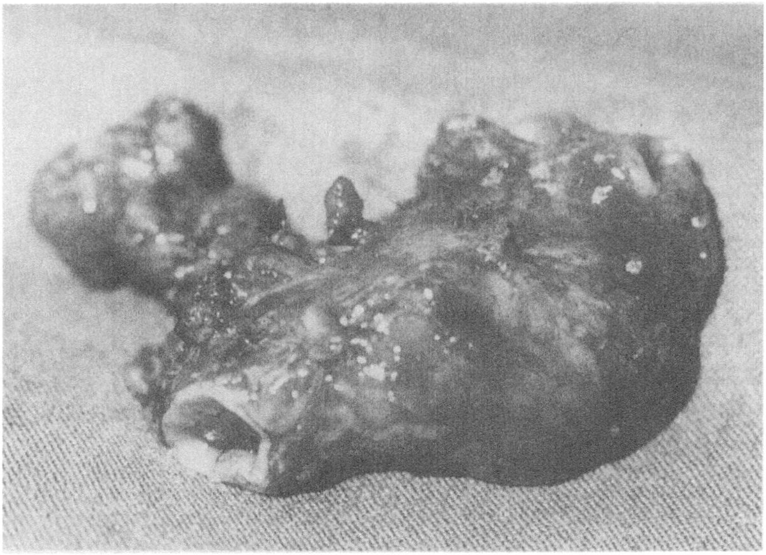

Fig. 2. Type III Klatskin tumor (adenocarcinoma, stage T1b) after resection. The dilated hepatic ducts are visible on the *right*, the small choledochus on the *left* side

resection in a standardized liver tissue-saving method [11] (Fig. 2). For radical excision, the resection had to be performed up to the secondary and tertiary convergencies of the hepatic ducts (Fig. 3). For bile flow reconstruction, we used stenting by silastic balloon catheters as shown in Figs. 4 and 5. The balloons were placed within at the previously prepared ROUX-en-Y bowel loop.

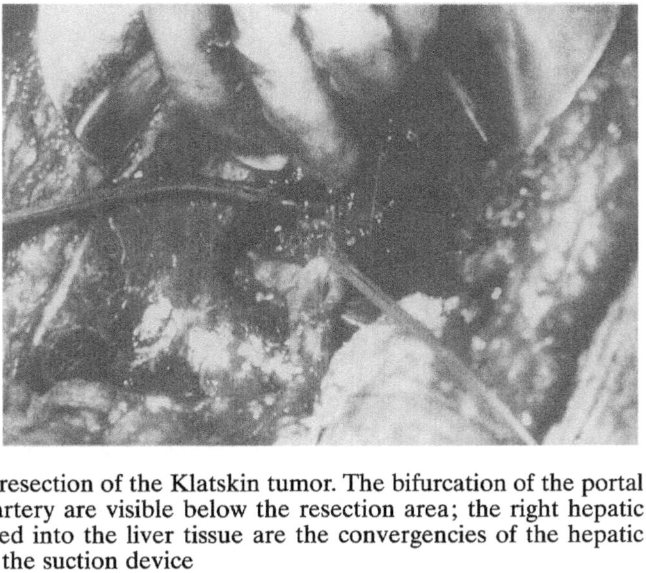

Fig. 3. Porta hepatis after resection of the Klatskin tumor. The bifurcation of the portal vein and the left hepatic artery are visible below the resection area; the right hepatic artery is resected. Retracted into the liver tissue are the convergencies of the hepatic ducts, as demonstrated by the suction device

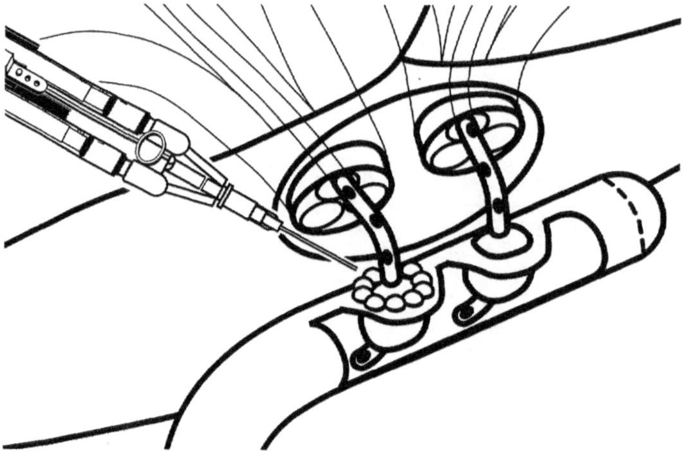

Fig. 4. Reconstruction of bile flow after resection of the hepatic bifurcation: silastic balloon catheters are placed into a Roux-en-Y loop serving as stent for the hepaticojejunostomy. Fixation of the anastomosis is performed by applying fibrin sealant only

The catheters, serving as inner and outer drainages, were pulled through the peripheral liver tissue as well as through the abdominal wall. By pulling the catheters, the bowel loop could be placed into the liver defect and approximated close to the peripheral hepatic ducts. Then, the catheters were fixed by a skin suture only, keeping the catheters under minimal tension. The fixation of the anastomosis itself was exclusively performed by a previously applied fibrin sealant (Fig. 4). This resulted in a totally sutureless anastomosis. Figure 6 demonstrates the end result of the bile flow reconstruction. Finally, the density of the anastomosis was proved by flushing the catheters with saline solution.

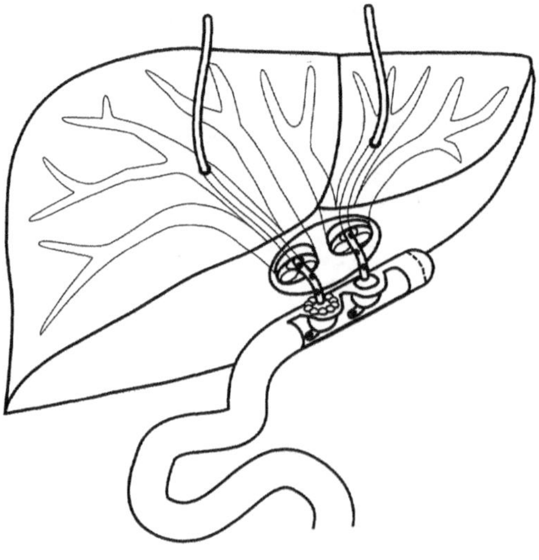

Fig. 5. Hepaticojejunostomy by fibrin sealing: after application of the fibrin sealant the loop is approximated onto the hepatic ducts by pulling the catheters only

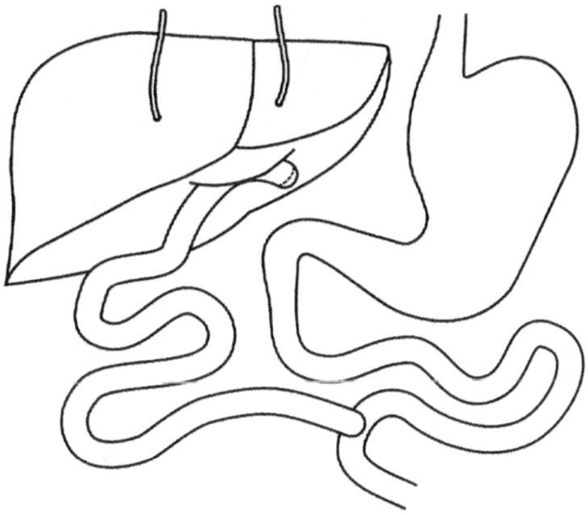

Fig. 6. Hepaticojejunostomy by fibrin sealing: final solution after the sealing; the catheters, pulled through the abdominal wall, are fixed by skin sutures only. They serve as short-term stenting and enable inner and outer bile drainage

A close postoperative follow-up of the patient was performed for 1 year postoperatively using laboratory liver function tests, ultrasonography, intravenous cholangiography, and Tc-99 m HIDA scintiscanning [11] for control.

Results

The postoperative outcome of the patient was without any complication. Laboratory liver function tests returned to normal within 2 weeks. The balloon catheters were used for short-term drainage and stenting only. They were removed on the 16 postoperative day, and the patient was dismissed from the hospital shortly after.

One year later, the patient was still fine and the liver function tests were within a normal range. Ultrasonography and intravenous cholangiogram revealed normal bile excretion (Fig. 7). To exclude any intrahepatic retention, we additionally investigated the patient by Tc-99 m HIDA scintiscanning as described by Iwasaky as the method for optimal proof [11]. The detailed sequence of normal excretion of the radioactive marker is shown in Fig. 8.

Discussion

After resection of the hepatic bifurcation, the surgeon is often confronted with a bleeding intrahepatic tissue surface, into which the secondary and tertiary convergencies of the bile ducts are retracted. Because of this and because of the lack of an appropriate visible exposition of the anastomotic sites during the anastomosing procedure, suturing of intrahepatic hepaticojejunostomy is far more difficult than is expressed by the usual schematas in operative textbooks. This situation is still reflected by a high operative mortality and a significant early and late complication rate, as initially mentioned.

Therefore, many attempts have been made during recent decades to facilitate bile flow reconstruction. One of the earliest attempts was to use transhe-

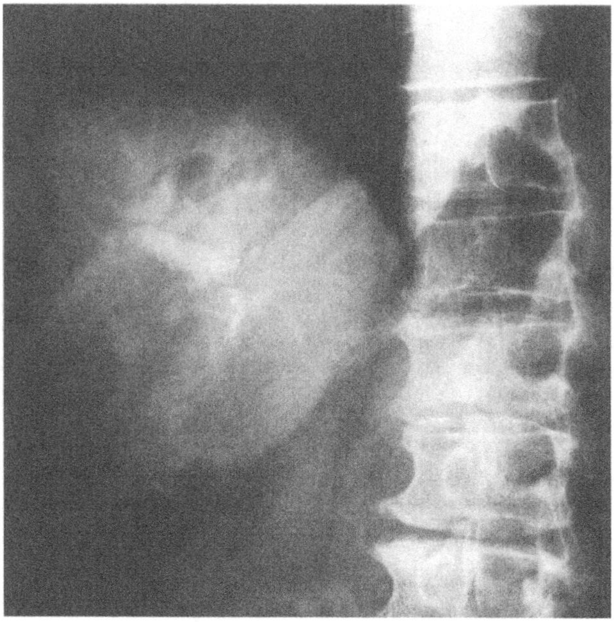

Fig. 7. Intravenous cholangiogram 1 year after hepaticojejunostomy: normal excretion of contrast medium. Intrahepatic ducts and the Roux-en-Y bowel loop are delineated; the blind end of the bowel loop is marked by the *staple line*

patic intubation for stenting of the anastomoses [10, 20]. This method allows sufficient bile drainage in even a less well-approximated and otherwise leaking anastomosis [7]; however, the less approximation of the anastomotic sites is achieved, the more scar formation and secondary stricture is likely to appear. Therefore, various authors recommend that stents are left for a longer period than that of a primary scar formation, such as up to 12 months and even longer [3, 6, 7, 23]. However, besides the inconvenience for the patient, long-term stenting and outer drainage favors infection and may lead to chronic cholangitis [4, 23].

As a further technical improvement, Wexler and Smith have suggested a "mucosal graft technique," pulling the Roux-en-Y loop up into the liver with the transhepatic tube [24]. The bowel wall is sutured to the liver capsula and only the bowel mucosa is sutured to the bile ducts or simply allowed to prolapse into the liver defect. Nevertheless, stenting seems to be necessary for 3–4 months and the success rate of only 65 % still does not indicate an optimal solution.

Furthermore, insufficient exposition of the deep-lying hepatic ducts seems to be the major technical problem. Therefore, extension of the resection itself as well has been used for a better exposition of the anastomotic sites. Bismuth advocates additional segment IV liver resection [2], while others have even tried a right or left hemihepatectomy [8, 9, 19]. Recent investigations by Lai and Tompkins demonstrated, however, that the mortality rate after such a liver

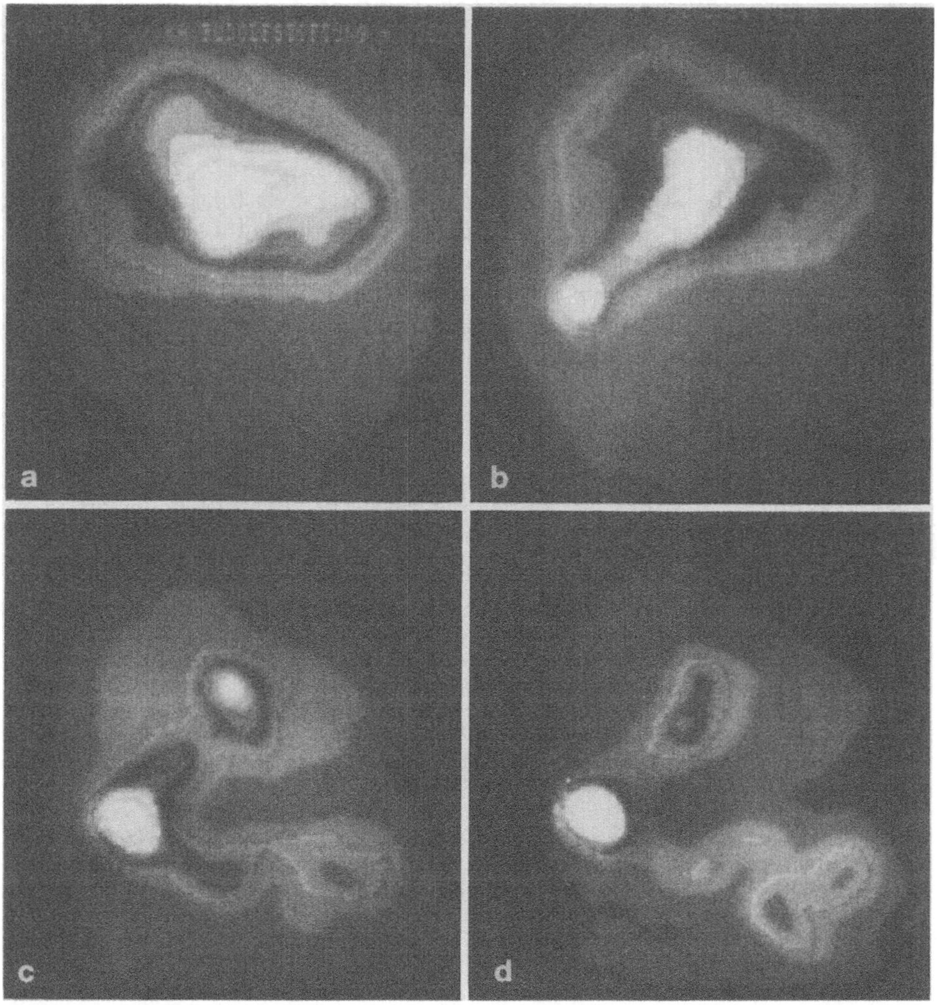

Fig. 8a–d. Tc-99 m HIDA scintiscanning 1 year after hepaticojejunostomy: sequence of excretion of the radioactive marker revealing normal bile flow through the blind loop into the small bowel within 2 h of administration

resection increased to 69 % whereas the long-term survival rate was not improved by radicality [13]. This seems to indicate that extended liver resection is not the appropriate way to overcome the technical problems.

Although the method we present in this chapter is simply a combination of preexisting techniques, it seems to be a significant step towards an optimal solution. On the one hand, the advanced technique of transhepatic intubation with silastic balloon catheters allows a tight mucosa-to-mucosa approximation of the anastomotic sites without any direct vision being necessary. The use of fibrin sealing on the other hand guarantees an immediately dense anastomosis without any danger of a minimal bile leakage or a resulting local inflammatory reaction followed by enhanced scar formation and secondary stenosis.

Conclusion

In our opinion, the advantages of our technique are as follows: First, it is a sutureless anastomosis, which can easily be performed in a standardized way and does not require special technical skill. Second, extended liver resection is not necessary. Optimal approximation of the anastomotic sites is possible and, finally, there seems to be only minor scar formation and a lower infection risk by using short-term stenting only.

References

1. Andersson A, Bergdahl L, van der Linden W (1977) Malignant tumors of the extrahepatic bile ducts. Surgery 81: 198–203
2. Bismuth H, Corlette MB (1975) Intrahepatic cholangioenteric anastomosis in carcinoma of the hilus of the liver. Surg Gynecol Obstet 140: 170–178
3. Block GE, Rosemurgy AS (1986) A technique for hepaticojejunostomy with transhepatic stent. Surg Gynecol Obstet 162: 485–487
4. Blumgart LH, Kelley CJ (1984) Hepaticojejunostomy in benign and malignant high bile duct stricture: approaches to the left hepatic ducts. Br J Surg 71: 257–261
5. Blumgart LH, Thompson JN (1987) The management of the malignant strictures of the bile duct. Curr Prob Surg 37: 88–93
6. Bolton JS, Braasch JW, Rossi RL (1980) Management of benign biliary stricture. Surg Clin North Am 60: 313–332
7. Cameron JL, Gayler BW, Zuidema GD (1978) The use of silastic transhepatic stents in benign and malignant biliary strictures. Ann Surg 188: 552–561
8. Evandon A, Fredlund P, Hoevels J, Ihse I, Bengmark S (1980) Evaluation of aggressive surgery in carcinoma of the extrahepatic bile ducts. Ann Surg 191: 23–27
9. Fortner JG, Kallum BO, Kim DK (1976) Surgical management of the main hepatic ducts. Ann Surg 184: 68–74
10. Goetze O (1951) Die transhepatische Dauerdrainage bei der hohen Gallengangsstenose. Arch Klin Chir 270: 97–102
11. Iwasaki Y, Okto M, Todoroky T (1977) Treatment of carcinoma of the biliary system. Surg Gynecol Obstet 144: 219–225
12. Klatskin G (1965) Adenocarcinoma of the hepatic duct at its bifurcation within the porta hepatis. Am J Med 38: 241–256
13. Lai ECS, Tompkins RK, Roslyn JJ, Mann LL (1987) Proximal bile duct cancer; quality of survival. Ann Surg 205: 111–118
14. Launois B, Campion JP, Brissot P, Gosselin M (1979) Carcinoma of the hepatic hilus. Ann Surg 190: 151–157
15. Longmire WP, McArthur MS, Bastounis EA (1973) Carcinoma of the extrahepatic biliary tract. Ann Surg 178: 333–337
16. Pellegrini CA, Thomas MJ, Way LW (1984) Recurrent biliary stricture. Am J Surg 147: 175–180
17. Pitt HA, Toshimitsus M, Parapatis SK, Tompkins RK, Longmire WP (1982) Factors influencing outcome in patients with postoperation biliary strictures. Am J Surg 144: 14–21
18. Ragins H, Diamond A, Meng CH (1973) Intrahepatic cholangiojejunostomy in the management of malignant biliary obstruction. Surg Gynecol Obstst 136: 27–31

19. Skoog V, Thoren L (1982) Carcinoma of the junctions of the main hepatic ducts. Acta Chir Scan 148: 411–415
20. Smith R (1964) Hepaticojejunostomy with transhepatic intubation. Br J Surg 51: 186–189
21. Terblanche J, Worthley CS, Spence RAJ, Krige JEJ (1990) High or low hepaticojejunostomy for bile duct strictures. Surgery 108: 828–834
22. Tompkins RK, Saunders KD, Roslyn JJ (1990) Changing patterns in diagnosis and management of bile duct cancer. Ann Surg 211: 614–621
23. Warren KW, Jefferson MF (1973) Prevention and repair of strictures of the extrahepatic bile ducts. Surg Clin North Am 53: 1169–1190
24. Wexler MJ, Smith R (1975) Jejunal mucosal graft: a sutureless technique for repair of high bilc duct strictures. Am J Surg 129: 204–206

Total Cystopericystectomy and Fibrin Sealant in the Treatment of Hydatid Disease of Liver

J. Hebrero San Martín and M. Fernández Ruiz

Abstract

We studied 267 cases of hydatid disease of the liver operated on in the last decade. Total removal of the cyst (cystectomy) was performed in 131 patients (49 %). In this group, 26 patients were included, in whom hepatic resection was added to the cystectomy as well as four who had biliobronchial fistula.

Some technical details of the surgical procedure and the management of biliobronchial fistula are described.

The wide cut surface of the liver after cystectomy was treated with fibrin sealant for the control of bleeding and biliary leaks, and this technique proved to be successful.

Postoperative complications were found in 19 % of patients, and only one patient died (mortality rate 0,7 %).

Indications and contraindications of this technique are revised and the efficacy of the fibrin sealant after cystectomy is stressed.

Introduction

Hydatid disease is still frequent in some areas of Spain, although it is decreasing slowly. Liver is the main location of the hydatid cyst, followed by lung, spleen, bones, and some other organs.

Surgical treatment is the only possible curative therapy for this disease, and indications for different operative techniques depend mainly on cyst size, number of cysts, their location in the liver, relationship with vascular and biliary main structure of the liver, and state and function of liver parenchyma.

As the main subjective of the operation is total eradication of the parasite and affected tissue of the liver, a radical removal of cyst and pericyst seems to be the best procedure, which must always be considered a major operation.

The main purpose of this report is to present the surgical technique proposed by the authors, its results, and some technical details.

Material and Methods

A consecutive series of 267 patients affected with hepatic hydatid cysts was studied and analyzed. The age range was 14–82 years and the mean age was 48 years. The male to female ratio was 1,3:1.

Solitary cysts were found in 161 patients (60.3 %) and multiple cysts in 106 (39.7 %; Fig. 1). In this series, there were cysts located in other organs besides the liver, such as lung and spleen in 42 patients (15.7 %).

A total of 157 patients (58.8 %) had total cystopericystectomy, some of them with some kind of hepatectomy added when necessary (group A), and 110 (41,2 %) had a less radical procedure: partial cystopericystectomy, simple cystectomy, aspiration drainage with external drainage, cystectomy, and omentoplasty (group B; Fig. 2).

Four patients in this series had cystopleural fistula, requiring a thoracic approach to remove part of either the right inferior or the middle lobe, and this maneuver was carried out as an extension of the primary procedure.

Operative Technique

The following steps must be carried out to perform a total cystopericystectomy:

1. An extended right subcostal incision provides good access in most patients.
2. Complete exposure of the lesion is needed and the number of cysts, their location in the liver and adhesions to other organs such as stomach, large bowel, and gallbladder have to be accurately assessed (Fig. 3). Continuous efforts must be made to evaluate the relation of the cysts with vascular and biliary structures.

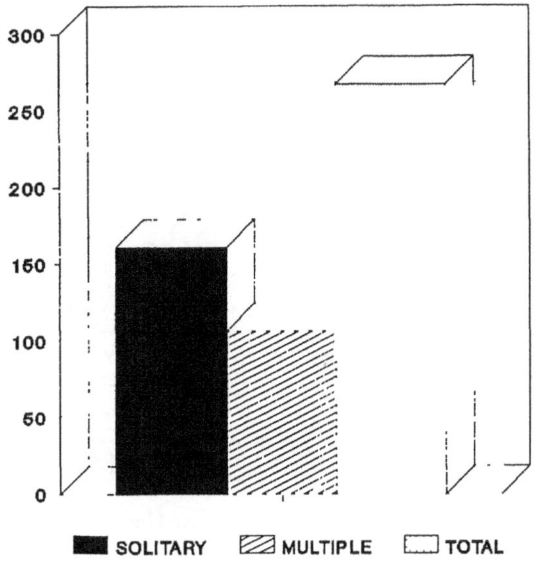

Fig. 1. Total number of patients in this series, and cases with solitary and multiple cysts

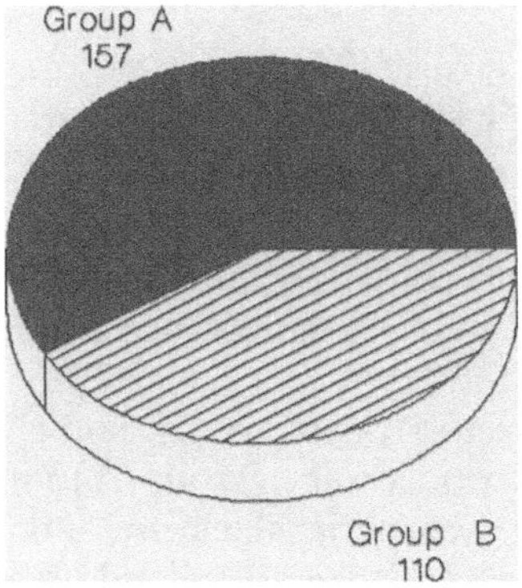

Fig. 2. Number of patients who had a radical total cystopericystectomy (group A) and patients with a nonradical, partial resection (group B)

3. An adequate dissection plane between pericyst and normal liver parenchyma must be found so that safe removal of the cyst can be carried out.
4. Conventional techniques for control of hemorrhage and bile leakage must be used. Blood vessels and biliary branches are handled by ligatures and sutures. Occasionally, a main suprahepatic vein has to be ligated and severed (Fig. 4).
5. A very large resection surface is left very often after total cystopericystectomy, depending on cyst size. Complete evaluation of this resection surface

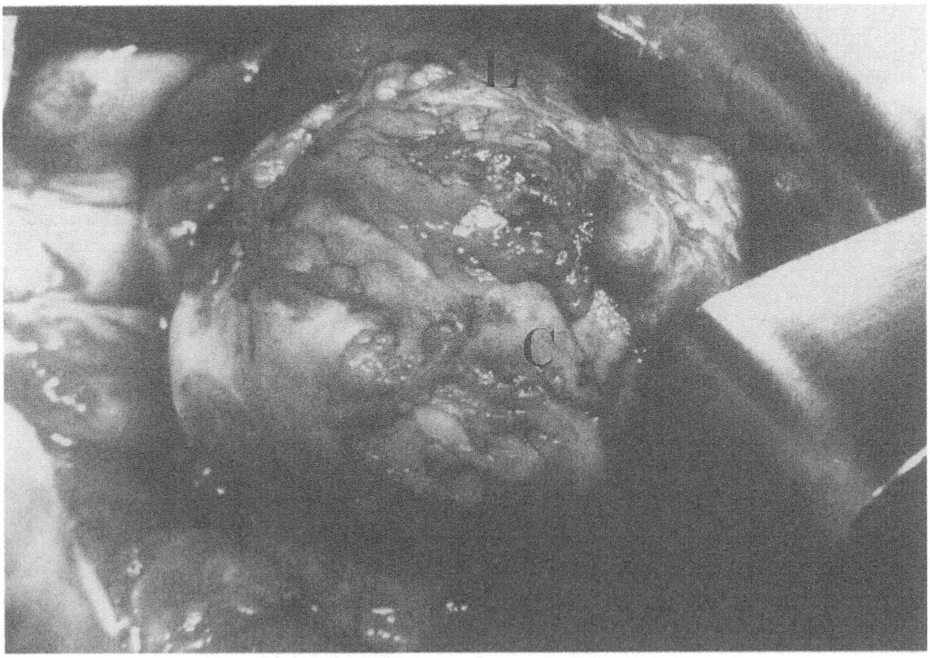

Fig. 3. Total cystopericystectomy. The cyst is being dissected free from the liver. *L*, Liver; *C*, cyst

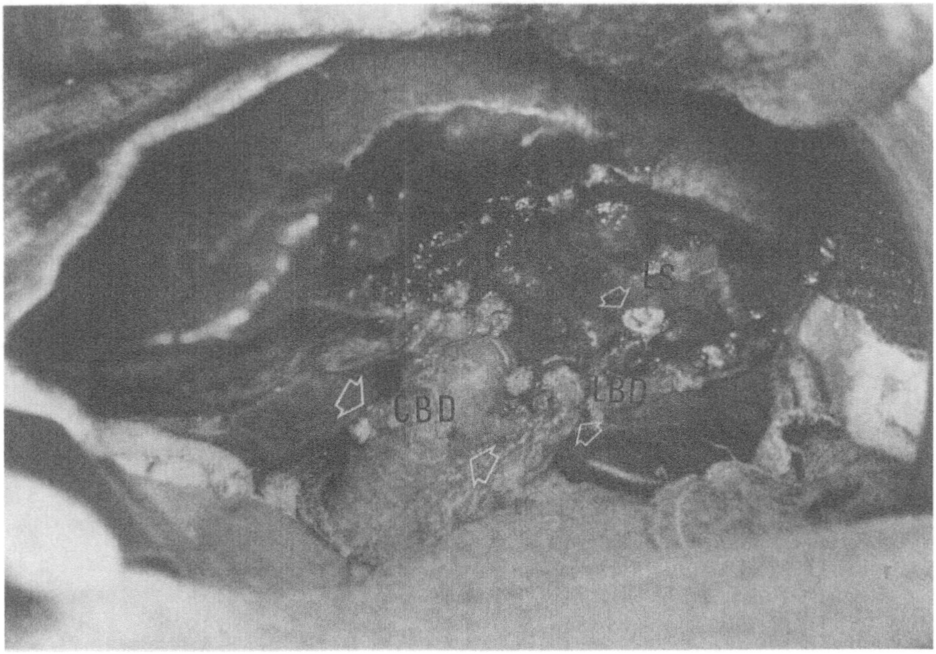

Fig. 4. A 15-cm cyst has been removed by left hemihepatectomy, and a cholecystectomy has been added. The common bile duct is dilated, the left biliary duct has been ligated and removed, and the left suprahepatic vein has been ligated and cut. *CBD*, Common bile duct; *LBD*, left biliary duct; *LS*, left suprahepatic vein

is needed, and any oozing hemorrhage and extravasation of bile must be carefully searched for (Fig. 5).

6. Adequate use of conventional hemostasis techniques is the precondition for treatment of bleeding and biliary leakage, but extravasation of blood and bile will persist in a significant number of cases. Fibrin sealant is applied to the resection surface of the liver for definitive control of any extravasation (Fig. 6).
7. External drainage is left in place for 4–9 days.

Advantages of Total Cystopericystectomy

Total cystopericystectomy is the only radical procedure by which the cyst is not opened during operation. On the contrary, it achieves complete radical removal of cyst contents and pericyst layer. There is no residual cavity left after the operation, as all diseased tissues are eliminated and only normal liver parenchyma remains. Complications linked to the residual cavity so often found with other surgical procedures do not arise with this operation.

Fewer biliary leakages and less bleeding complicate the operation, as every biliary branch and blood vessel can be easily identified, isolated, and ligated on

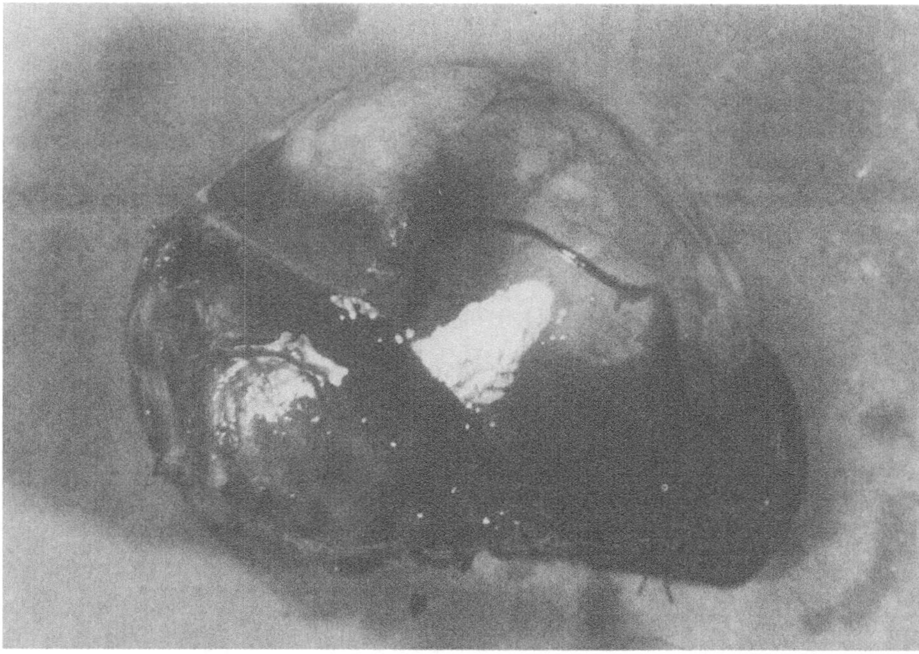

Fig. 5. Large cyst removed from left hepatic lobe

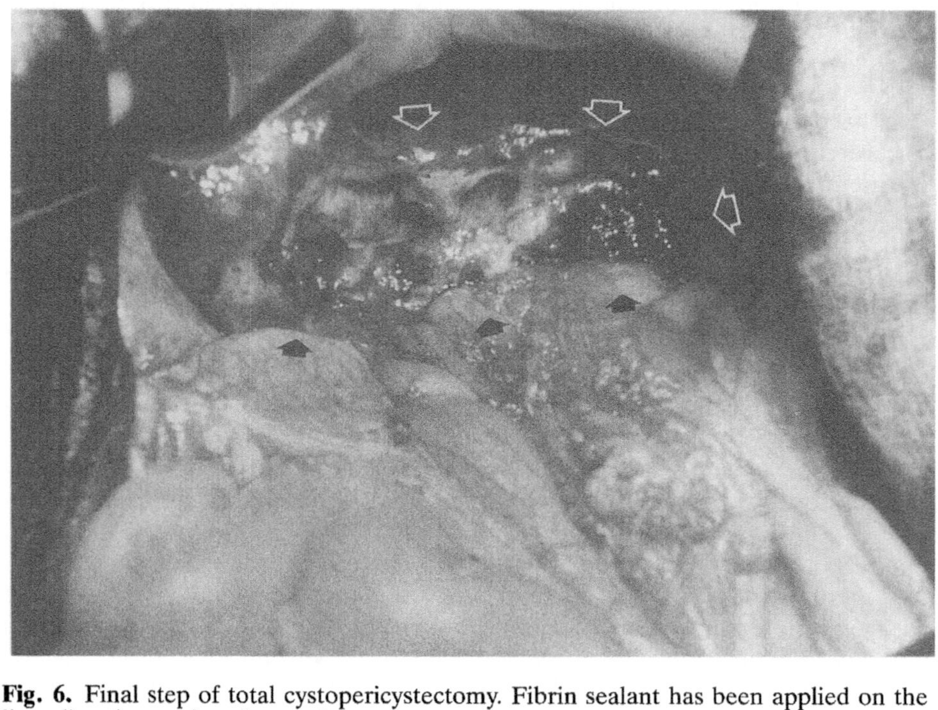

Fig. 6. Final step of total cystopericystectomy. Fibrin sealant has been applied on the liver disection surface *(arrows)*

the extracystic plane. Fibrin sealant can be applied on the raw liver resection surface, thus diminishing both active bleeding and postoperative biliary leakage. Cyst recurrences are avoided, as total cystopericystectomy completely eliminate both the disease and the possibility of further spreading due to intraoperative maneuvers.

Results

Hospital stay was shorter in group A (13 days) than in group B (19.8 days). No patient died in group A (0%) and two died in group B (1.8%), the total mortality rate being 0.7%. There were postoperative complications in group A in 21 patients (13%) and in group B in 23 (26%) (Table 1).

Postoperative biliary fistulae occurred in 19 cases out of the total series of 267 patients and endoscopic-sphincterotomy was needed in nine of these.

Conclusions

The surgical technique described in this paper offers several unique advantages:

- Total cystopericystectomy has proved to be very effective and safe as surgical treatment of hydatid disease of the liver.
- Fibrin sealant applied on the resection liver surface is very useful to achieve complete control of hemorrhage and biliary leakage.
- With this technique, there is less morbidity and mortality and recurrences are avoided.

Table 1. Postoperative complications

	Group A	Group B
External fistulae	4	6
Hemorrhage	3	5
Subphrenic abscess	1	2
Abdominal abscess	1	1
Sepsis	1	2
Respiratory failure	1	1
Wound infection	4	3
Pleural effusion	4	2
Pneumonia	2	–
Pulmonary embolism	–	1
Total	21 (13%)	23 (20%)

References

1. Akoglu M, Davidson BR (1992) A rational approach to the terminology of hydatid disease of the liver. J. Infect 24 (1): 1–6
2. Belghiti J, Perniceni T, Kabbej M, Fekete F (1991) Complications of preoperative sterilization of hydatid cysts of the liver. Apropos of 6 cases, Chirurgie 117 (5–6): 343–346
3. Bossi L, del Corno G (1990) Diagnostic and therapeutic of human hydatidosis. Study of a hospital case series. Parassitologia 32 (3): 363–369
4. Cangiotti L, Giulini SM, Muiesan P, Nodari F, Begni A, Tiberio G (1991) Hydatid disease of the liver: long term results of surgical treatment. G Chir 12 (10): 501–504
5. Elhamel A (1990) Pericystectomy for the treatment of hepatic hydatid cysts. Surgery 107 (3): 316–320
6. Magistrelli P, Masetti R, Coppola R, Messia A, Nuzzo G, Picciocchi A (1991) Surgical treatment of hydatid disease of the liver. A 20-year experience. Arch Surg 126 (4): 518–522
7. Mentha G, Morel P, Buhler L, Huber O, Klopfenstein CE, Rohner A (1991) Surgical treatment of hepatic hydatidosis. Schweiz Med Wochenschr 121 (35): 1231–1237
8. Moreno Gonzáles E, Rico Selas P, Martínez B, Garcia Garcia I, Palma Carazo F, Hidalgo Pascual M (1991) Results of surgical treatment of hepatic hydatidosis: current therapeutic modifications. World J Surg 15 (2): 254–263
9. Movchun AA, Koloss OE, Shatverian GA, Abdullaev AG, Alikhanov NKh (1991) Errors and hazards in the surgical treatment of hepatic echinococcosis. Khirurgiia (Mosk). 11: 113–117
10. Ozmen V, Igci A, Kebudi A et al (1992) Surgical treatment of hepatic hydatid disease. Can J Surg 35 (4): 423–427
11. Vignote ML, Miño G, de la Mata M, de Dios JF, Gómez F (1990) Endoscopic sphincterotomy in hepatic hydatid disease open to the biliary tree. Br J Surg 77 (1): 30–31
12. Xynos E, Pechlivanides G, Tzortzinis A, Papageorgiou A, Vassilakis JS (1991) Hydatid disease of the liver. Diagnosis and surgical treatment. HPB Surg 4 (1): 59–66

Indications for Fibrin Sealing in Pancreatic Surgery with Special Regard to Occlusion of a Nonanastomosed Stump with Fibrin Sealant

A. P. Marczell

Abstract

In surgery of the pancreas, the rate of complications is high due to the specific properties of pancreatic surgery. A report on a new method, used in over 200 cases, proves that fibrin sealant can significantly reduce the complication rate; especially in the Whipple procedure for malignancies, results were improved by occlusion of the pancreatic stump with fibrin sealant.

Among 67 patients treated with this method, there were no perioperative deaths and four patients developed local complications (three fistulae, one pancreatitis) due to technical errors that presumably resulted in incomplete occlusion. The long-term results with regard to endocrine function are satisfactory.

Introduction

Pancreatic surgery is generally accompanied by a high complication rate. Due to the specific properties of pancreatic tissue, sutures of the parenchyma lead to ischemic necroses, which in turn become foci of inflammation resulting in typical local complications such as postoperative hemorrhage, persistent pancreatitis, and pancreatic fistulae. It is interesting that even after so-called minor interventions the complication rate is high (Table 1).

Table 1. Average complication and mortality rates

	Complication rate (%)	Mortality rate (%)
Biopsy or wedge resection	9.5	3.8
Enucleation	0.0–43	4.5–13
Tail resection or extended left pancreatectomy	0.0–41	1.0–11
Whipple's operation	16.4–44	4.5–23 (36.6)
Internal drainage	27.0	6.1
Trauma	25.0–75.0	?

Applications of Fibrin Sealant

The generally poor results – except in single consecutive series [1–3] – were the reason we have applied fibrin sealant increasingly in pancreatic surgery in the following indications:

Wedge Excisions and Enucleations

The rate of complications in wedge excisions and with enucleation methods is reported to be up to 23 % [4, 5], mainly due to pancreatic fistulae, with which the mortality rate is 4.5 %–6,2 % [5]. Fibrin sealing allows seamless sealing of the tissue defect. In this case, the defect is filled up or packed with the sealant without any suturing. We have treated more than 30 patients by this method and have observed no postoperative complications.

Tail Resections and Extended Left Pancreatectomy

Even at hospitals that are not specialized in pancreatic surgery, it is often necessary to manage resection surfaces or extensive superficial tissue defects of the pancreas parenchyma, e.g., in extended gastrectomies with lymph node dissection, in carcinomata of the left flexure, or in traumatic lesions. Also after splenectomies of large spleens for hematological reasons it may be necessary to treat lesions of the pancreatic tail. After interventions of this type, the complication rate is as high as 41 % [5], pancreatic fistulae accounting for two thirds of these problems. The mortality rate is relatively high, too, ranging from 4.3 % to 11 % [6, 7].

The operative sealing method is as follows: superficial lesions are sealed like anastomoses, whereas deep defects, such as wedge excisions, are packed with the sealant.

Following tail resection or left pancreatectomy without an exposable pancreatic duct, the resection surface is trimmed in the form of a fish mouth, the gaping wound edges are approximated and sealed, and the "lips" are covered with an additional coat of the fibrin sealant.

Even in extensive, recently performed left pancreatectomy, we have found only two cases of postoperative complications (pancreatic fistulae).

Partial Pancreatectomy (Whipple Procedure): Occlusion of a Nonanastomosed Pancreatic Stump with Fibrin Sealant

Following Whipple's operation for chronic pancreatitis, both anastomoses are sealed imperviously with fibrin sealant. By this method excellent results can be achieved [8].

Following partial pancreatectomy (PDP) for malignant indication, the complication and mortality rates are particularly high (Table 2). The average

Table 2. Perioperative complication and mortality rates associated with pancreaticoduodenectomy for malignant indication

Author	Year	Complications (%)	Mortality (%)
Schapiro [9]	1975	50	8
Nakase [10]	1977	49	21
Warren [11]	1983		
	(1951–1960)	–	14
	(1971–1980)	–	3.4
Kümmerle and Rückert [12]	1984	–	20
van Heerden [13]	1984	33	4
Grace et al. [14]	1986		
	(1975–1979)	49	10
	(1980–1984)	26	2
Tarazi et al. [15]	1986	40	7
Christ et al. [16]	1987		
	(1969–1980)	59	24
	(1981–1986)	36	2
Trede and Schwall [17]	1988	32	3

perioperative mortality rate cited for Whipple's procedure has been around 14%, with a range between 3% and 24%, and postoperative complications have been observed in almost half the patients. However, in the past decade morbidity and mortality rates have been falling [7, 11, 13, 14, 16, 18].

The poor results seen following PDP are due largely to leakage from the pancreaticoenteric anastomoses, infection, or postoperative hemorrhage from the upper gastrointestinal tract or the resection site [11, 13, 14, 16]. In cases of chronic pancreatitis these complications do not appear, due to progressive sclerosis and the coarse capsule of the pancreas.

A variety of surgical techniques have been tried in order to reduce the incidence of postoperative complications, with particular emphasis on decreasing the incidence of pancreatic fistulas resulting from the lytic effects of pancreatic enzymes on the pancreaticojejunostomy.

The methods tried have been: (a) open management stump [19], (b) ligation, (c) splinting (stenting) of the pancreatic duct [20], and (d) various anastomosis techniques and occlusion [4, 21]. Occlusion with synthetic materials such as prolamine (Ethibloc [4]) and neoprene have been used in both pancreatic cancer and transplantation surgery with reported success in blocking the pancreatic ductal system, but with evidence of occasional transient pancreatic fistulas and/or progressive failure of pancreatic endocrine function due to progressive sclerosis.

A desire to decrease morbidity and mortality due to leakage at pancreaticojejunal anastomoses led us to evaluate an atraumatic, sutureless method for pancreatic stump management – stump occlusion with a physiologic agent that we hoped would not elicit foreign body reaction in the pancreatic stump and subsequent fibrosis of the remaining gland with damage to the islets.

Method

Following Whipple's resection, the remaining ducts were occluded with fibrin sealant. Approximately 3–5 ml fibrin sealant was injected into the main pancreatic duct, either through a blunt needle or a thin plastic catheter, beginning as deeply as possible in the remaining glandular tissue. As the needle or catheter is slowly withdrawn, fibrin sealant is continuously injected until small fibrin thrombi appear on the resection surface. The pancreatic duct is then ligated and the resection area is covered with an additional layer of sealant. Collagen fleece may be applied if hemorrhage is difficult to control (Figs. 1–4). This method was employed in 67 patients (38 male, 29 female) undergoing partial pancreaticoduodenectomy for malignancy. There were 12 patients with carcinoma of the common bile duct, 20 with papillary carcinoma, and 35 patients with carcinoma of the head of the pancreas. The average age was 67,5 years and 76 % of the patients were older than 70 years.

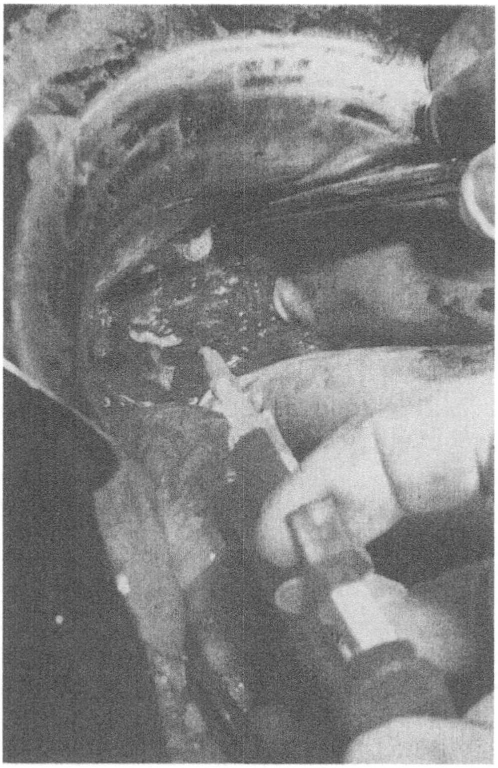

Fig. 1. Duct occlusion with fibrin sealant

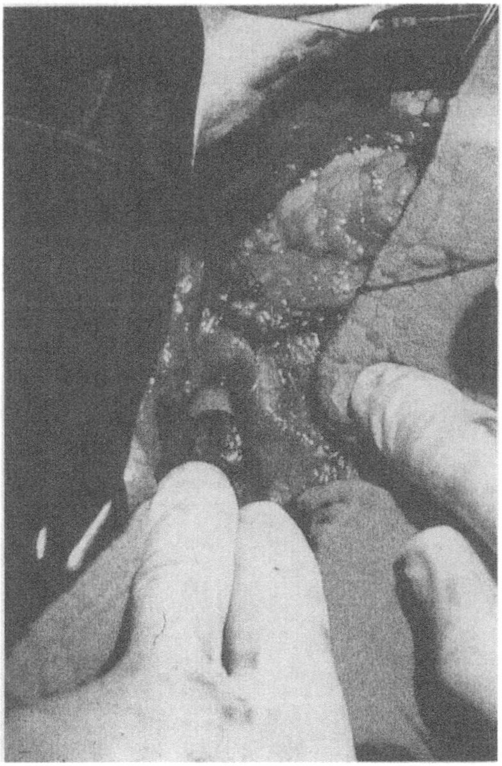

Fig. 2. Ligature of the occluded duct

Results

There were no perioperative deaths among the 67 patients. One patient developed clinical evidence of persistent necrotizing pancreatitis, necessitating total pancreatectomy. Three patients developed pancreatic fistulas, probably caused by incomplete occlusion; with conservative therapy, these receded within 2–4 weeks postsurgery. Technical shortcomings in these four patients treated early in our series probably led to incomplete occlusion and, as a consequence, persistent pancreatitis.

In all patients, we noted a moderate elevation of amylase levels in both serum and urine, which subsided after 1 week. To compensate for the loss of pancreatic enzymes, all surviving patients were given pancreatic granules as a dietary supplement.

With regard to pancreatic endocrine function, all the patients with normal glucose tolerance before surgery were unchanged postoperatively. Among those patients with latent diabetes, demonstrated by abnormal preoperative glucose tolerance tests, 20 % developed manifest diabetes postsurgery. Among these patients, the manifest diabetes can be attributed to resection of intact pancreatic tissue.

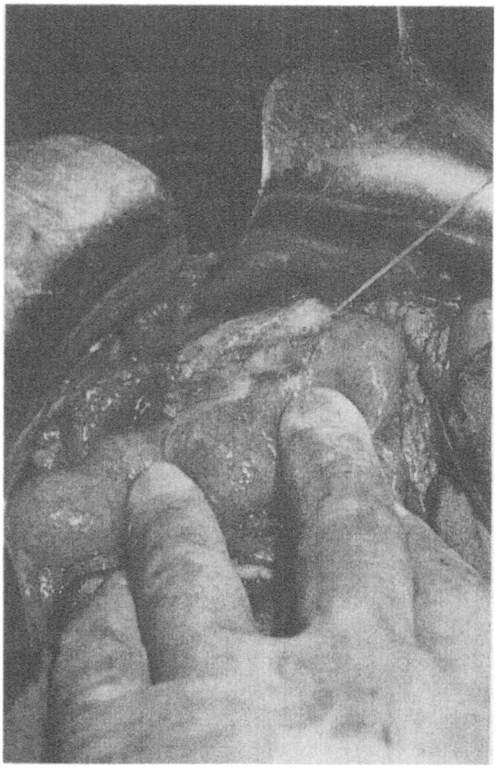

Fig. 3. Sealing of the resection surface with fibrin sealant

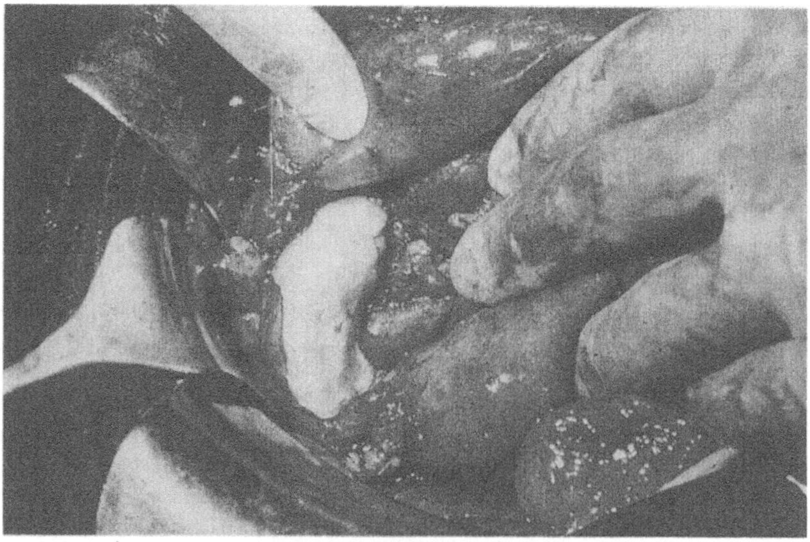

Fig. 4. Sealing in combination with collagen fleece

After an observation period of 4½ years, 21 of the surviving patients had normal fasting blood sugar levels; six of these patients had normal fasting blood sugar after 5 years.

Internal Drainage

In interventions to secure internal drainage, the anastomosis can be sealed with a cuff of fibrin sealant, possibly also on the inside, to prevent not only insufficiencies, but also arrosion bleeding [22].

Traumatic Lesions

In cases of traumatic lesions, the rate of complications and that of mortality depend on the extent of the lesion. This explains the divergent figures reported in the literature. Depending on the severity of the lesion, postoperative complications are expected in 25 %–75 % cases, most frequently with pancreatic fistulae. In my opinion, it is advisable to use fibrin sealant for the following indications: (a) lesions of the tail, possibly perforating; (b) combined head and corpus lesions with intact main duct; and (c) management of all resection surfaces.

Discussion

In 241 applications of fibrin sealant, we have had only 12 failures (Table 3).

Comparative studies by Ascherl and his Munich team [23] showed that fibrin sealant is best suited for pancreas occlusion; due to its low viscosity, it is superior to other occlusion media such as prolamin. Additional advantages are its hemostatic and its fluidtight sealing effect, which are particularly useful in this organ.

Table 3. Applications and results of fibrin sealing in the pancreas

	n	Local failures
Biopsy	28	1
Enucleation	10	0
Lymph node dissection	58	1
Tail resection or left pancreatectomy	42	2
Head resection	10	1[a]
Head resection with duct occlusion	67	4[b]
Drainage operations	16	0
Traumatic lesions	10	3
Total	241	12[a]

[a] Lethality.
[b] Total pancreatectomy has to be performed.

The high fibrinolytic activity of pancreatic tissue requires high aprotinin concentration of the sealant (at least 10000 kIU/ml) to avoid premature dissolution of fibrin. Especially in minor interventions on the pancreas, our results are satisfactory. This is interesting inasmuch as these operations can be performed not only at specialized clinics, but also in general hospitals. Here, fibrin sealant certainly helps to reduce the complication rate.

Fibrin occlusion has also led to improved postoperative results after Whipple's operation by using this low-viscosity agent. Occlusion of the pancreatic duct with prolamin does not yield uniformly favorable long-term results, probably because the high and variable viscosity of this material hampers complete occlusion of the collateral branches [23]. Furthermore, occlusion with prolamin in usually followed by interstitial fibrosis with subsequent high-grade sclerosis of the exocrine pancreatic parenchyma beginning on the second postoperative day, with significant alteration of the endocrine cell relation [24].

Occlusion with fibrin sealant could significantly reduce perioperative mortality as well as the postoperative complication rate of partial pancreaticoduodenectomy by employing fibrin sealant occlusion of the remaining pancreatitis ducts, and we are continuing to see satisfactory long-term results, certainly due to less interstitial reaction and fibrosis of this physiologic substance, which does not induce a foreign body reaction. Simple handling and the atraumatic approach justify routine use of this method.

References

1. Bodner E (1981) Chirurgie des Pankreas: Das Pankreaskarzinom. Acta Chir Austriaca 13: 94
2. Hicks RE, Brooks JR (1971) Total pancreatectomy for ductal carcinoma. Surg Gynecol Obstet 133: 16
3. Trede M, Hoffmeister AW (1982) Chirurgische Therapie des Pankreaskarzinoms. Therapiewoche 32: 918
4. Gebhardt C, Stolte M (1978) Die Ausschaltung des exkretorischen Pankreasparenchyms durch intraduktale Injektion einer schnell härtenden Aminosäurelösung. Chirurg 49: 428
5. Spelsberg F, Heberer G, Landgraf R, Wirsching R (1978) Klinik, Diagnostik und Behandlung des organischen Hyperinsulinismus. Munch Med Wochenschr 120: 547
6. Frick S (1982) Komplikationen nach resezierenden Eingriffen bei chronischer Pankreatitis. Langenbecks Arch Chir 356: 82
7. Rückert K., Kümmerle F (1979) Das Papillenca. Chirurg 50: 308
8. Scheele J (1982) Klinische Erfahrungen mit der Fibrinklebung an parenchymatösen Oberbauchorganen. Aktuel Chir 17: 153
9. Schapiro TM (1975) Adenocarcinoma of the pancreas: a statistical analysis of biliary bypass vs Whipple resection in good risk patients. Ann Surg 182: 715–721
10. Nakase A, Honjo I, Matsumoto Y, Uchida K (1977) Surgical treatment of cancer of the pancreas and the periampullary region. Ann Surg 185: 52
11. Warren KW, Armendariz R, Basu S, Christoph C (1983) Current trends in the diagnosis and treatment of carcinoma of the pancreas. Am J Surg 145: 813–818
12. Kümmerle F, Rückert K (1984) Surgical treatment of pancreatic cancer. World J Surg 8: 889–894
13. Van Heerden JA (1984) Pancreatic resection for carcinoma of the pancreas: whipple versus total pancreatectomy – an institutional perspective. World J Surg 8: 880–888

14. Grace PA, Denbentsen L, Longmire WP, Pitt HA, Tompkins RK (1986) Decreased morbidity and mortality after pancreatoduodenoectomy. Am J Surg 151: 141–148
15. Tarazi RY, Esselstyn jr CB, Hermann RE, Hoerr SO, Vogt DP (1986) Results of surgical treatment of periampullary tumors: a thirty-five-year experience. Surgery 100: 716–722
16. Christ DW, Cameron JL, Sitzmann JV (1987) Improved hospital morbidity, mortality, and survival after the Whipple procedure. Ann Surg 206: 358–365
17. Trede M, Schwall G (1988) The complications of pancreatectomy. Ann Surg 207: 39–47
18. Warshaw AL, Swanson RS (1988) Pancreatic cancer in 1988. Possibilities and probabilities. Ann Surg 208: 541–552
19. Funovics 3, Wenzl E (1985) Duodenopankreatektomie: Anastomosierung nicht notwendig. Langenbecks Arch Chir 366: 613
20. Schopohl J, Droese K, Zöckler CE (1986) Ein modifiziertes Whipple'sches Operationsverfahren. Chirurg 57: 517
21. Marczell A (1986) The use of Tissucol in pancreatic surgery. In: Schlag G, Redl W (eds) General surgery and abdominal surgery. Springer, Berlin Heidelberg New York, p 140 (Fibrin sealant in operative medicine, vol 6)
22. Zirngibl H, Faszbender D, Gebhardt C (1983) Drainagebehandlung von Pankreaspseudozysten. Langenbecks Arch Chir 360: 19
23. Ascherl R, Blümel G, Geissdörfer K, Hirmer H, Richling B (1985) Pankreasgangokklusion mit Fibrin, 102nd Meeting of the Deutsche Gesellschaft für Chirurgie
24. Grossner D, Berkhoff M, Klapder F, Klöppel G, Von Koge H (1989) Insulinreserve und Morphologie des Pankreasschwanzes nach Pankreaskopfresektion bei unterschiedlichen Methoden der Versorgung. Langenbecks Arch Chir 374: 4–11

The Application of Fibrin Sealant in Pancreatic Surgery

K. HIRATA, T. MIKAMI, I. OIKAWA, T. KATSURAMAKI, K. YAMASIRO, M. MUKAIYA, A. OKAZAKI, H. KIMURA, K. SASAKI, and R. DENNO

Abstract

Well-controlled comparative studies with or without fibrin sealant were conducted to evaluate (a) the effect on prevention of anastomotic insufficiency of pancreaticojejunostomy and (b) the effect on the sealing of small ducts and vessels in the resected surface of the pancreas. A total of 36 patients who had undergone pancreaticojejunostomy were examined, i.e., 16 cases treated with fibrin sealant in anastomosis and 20 cases treated without. A total of 20 cases of distal pancreatectomy were also examined, i.e., ten cases treated with and ten cases treated without fibrin sealant in the resected surface.

The incidence of anastomotic insufficiency was one in 16 with fibrin sealant (6.3 %) and three in 20 without (15.0 %); hence, there was a small difference between the two groups. The total incidence of bacterial infection with partial tissue necrosis was one in 16 with (6.3 %) and three in 20 without fibrin sealant (15.0 %). Thus, there was a small difference here as well.

In addition, the small amount of leakage of pancreatic juice from the resected surface with or without low-grade infection was studied. The incidences were one in ten with and one in ten without fibrin sealant; hence, no difference was observed between the two groups in this operation.

These data indicate the lower incidences of local complications in relation to most earlier reports and the effectiveness of fibrin sealant in the prevention of leakage of pancreatic juice and for hemostasis.

Introduction

It is well known that after pancreatectomy, the incidence of local complications, e.g., leakage of pancreatic juice, anastomotic insufficiency, and intra-abdominal abscess, is still high [6, 8]. The most distressing problem in these complications is the occurrence of serious conditions which might lead to operative death in some patients. Such conditions are mainly caused by incorrect drainages in addition to the complication. Accordingly, it is very important to concentrate on positioning drainage tubes accurately just before closure of the peritoneum. Otherwise, these complications may be induced due to incomplete hemostasis or the small breakdown of anastomosis. Therefore, in order to avoid serious complications in the early stages after an operation, strict handling in pancreatojejunostomy is necessary, especially in pancreatoduodenectomy. Moreover, it would be helpful to have materials which protect against the occurrence of anastomotic insufficiency or minor bleeding. Even when experienced surgeons perform pancreatoduodenectomy, it is very difficult for all procedures during an operation to be performed completely. Fibrin sealants have recently been introduced to achieve hemostasis and/or better healing processes [4, 5]. There have not been many reports about its effect on the healing process in the resected surface after pancreatectomy [3, 10]. In this study, we tried to clinically verify two kinds of effects of fibrin sealants: (1) their effect on the prevention of anastomotic insufficiency in pancreaticojejunostomy and (2) their effect on hemostasis around a pancreaticojejunostomy or the resected surface and on the prevention of juice leakage from small pancreatic ducts in the resected surface.

Materials and Methods

Patients and Study Method

This clinical study was carried out by retrospective analysis and was open to patients from January 1987 to December 1991. Thirty-six patients with a malignancy of the pancreatoduodenal region and 20 patients with resectable gastric carcinoma were registered. The patients in the former group underwent pancreatoduodenectomy with or without pyrolus preservation and the patients in the latter group underwent distal pancreatectomy with splenectomy or dissect parapancreatic lymph nodes around splenic vessels. In each group, patients were then assigned to two subgroups; in one, fibrin sealants were used and in the other, they were not (Table 1).

Operation Method

The fundamental idea concerning pancreatoduodenectomy in our department should first be introduced. It is necessary to realize that the healing process after pancreaticojejunostomy may be impaired, due to possible microscopical tissue destruction, metabolic disturbance, and the low biological response,

Table 1. Randomized prospective study on the effects of fibrin sealant after pancreatectomy

Treatment after pancreatectomy	Fibrin sealant		Total
	(+)	(–)	
Pancreaticojejunostomy	16	20	36
Pancreatectomy	10	10	20

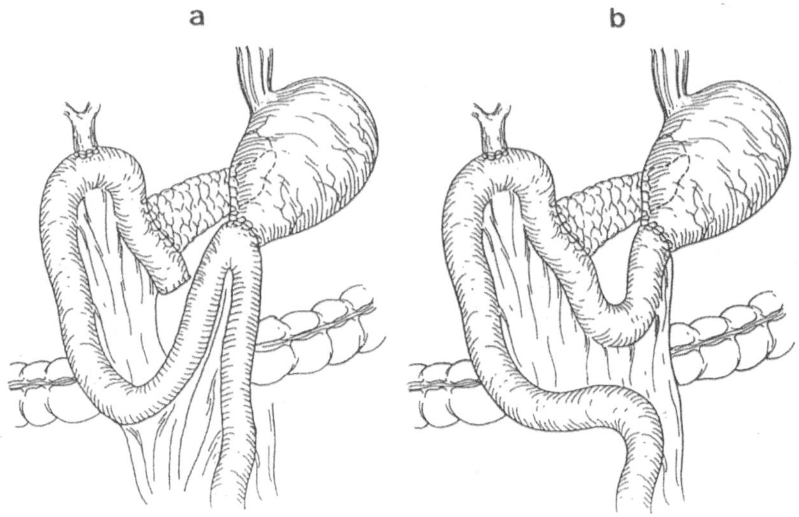

Fig. 1 a, b. Methods of reconstruction. **a** Child's method (modified). **b** Imanaga's method

because we usually perform extended radical operations, which involve the dissection of regional lymph nodes distributed in the parapancreatoduodenal region and in the bilateral para-aortic region between the diaphragm and the right renal vein. Moreover, two thirds of the celiac plexus in the lesion side are resected. Reconstructions were performed by the modified Child's method (Fig. 1a) for elderly patients or patients with severe coexistent disease, e.g. severe metabolic disease and severe cardiopulmonary diseases, and by Imanaga's method (Fig. 1b) for younger patients who underwent complete curative operations. End-to-side anastomosis in pancreaticojejunostomy was employed in all cases (Fig. 2).

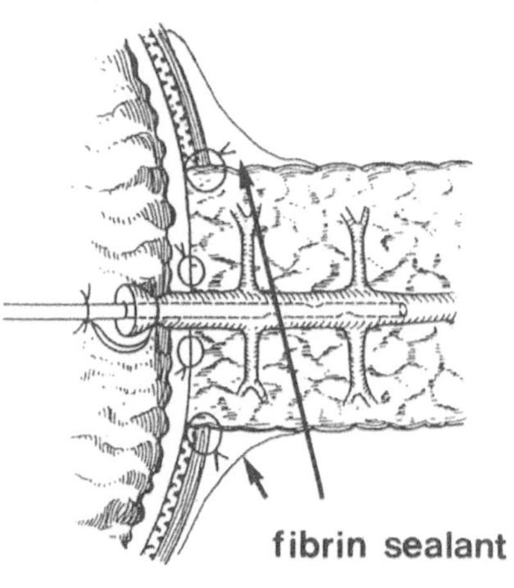

Fig. 2. End-to-side anastomosis in pancreaticojejunostomy

As to the drainage, tube insertion into main pancreatic duct was surely settled out. Moreover, only in patients with a dilated pancreatic duct was anastomosis between the main pancreatic duct and jejunal mucosa carried out; in patients with no dilatation of the pancreatic duct, the main pancreatic duct was used for fixation of the drainage tube, because an anastomosis between the pancreatic duct and the jejunal mucosa is difficult technically and can easily leak if the pancreas has a soft consistency and the main pancreatic duct is small. After drainage, suture of the pancreatic parenchyma and the seromuscular layer of the jejunum and of the seroparenchyma of the pancreas and the seromuscular layer of the jejunum was carried out using nylon twine and monofilamentous nylon threads, respectively. Fibrin sealant was employed around the pancreaticojejunostomy. In distal pancreatectomy, the main pancreatic duct was ligated, hemostasis was achieved using 6–0 monofilamentous nylon thread, and fibrin sealant was applied in order to manage the resected surface of pancreas.

Results

Comparison of Risk Factors

In pancreatoduodenectomy, there were no significant differences in age, condition of the pancreatic duct and parenchyma, reconstruction method used, or frequency of malignancy as the primary disease (Table 2). In distal pancreatectomy, there were also no significant differences in age, condition of the pancreas, or frequency of malignancy. However, the number of males was higher in the fibrin sealant subgroup of patients undergoing the latter operation.

Table 2. Cox's multiregression model of risk factors for patients with pancreaticobiliary disease

	Pancreaticojejunostomy	Distal pancreatectomy
	(–)[a] (+)[b]	(–)[a] (+)[b]
Age	N. S.	N. S.
Sex	N. S.	$p<0.05$
Pancreas		
Dilatation of MPD	N. S.	N. S.
Fibrosis (–)	N. S.	N. S.
(+)	N. S.	N. S.
Reconstruction method		
Child	N. S.	–
Imanaga	N. S.	–
Malignancy	N. S.	N. S.

MPD, main pancreatic duct; N. S., not significant.
[a] Fibrin glue not used.
[b] Fibrin glue used.

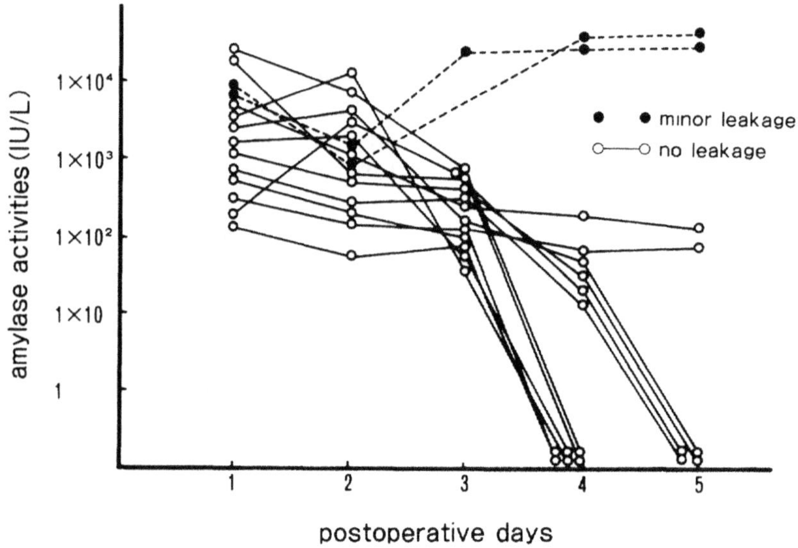

Fig. 3. Changes in amylase activities in fluid draining into the perianastomosis of pancreaticojejunostomy in patients without fibrosis of the pancreas

Changes in Amylase Activities in Fluid Draining into the Perianastomosis

In patients without fibrosis in the pancreas, amylase activities in the fluid draining into the perianastomosis of pancreatojejunostomy were quantified for 5 days after pancreatoduodenectomy. As shown in Fig. 3, amylase activities rapidly decreased during the 3 postoperative days in patients without leakage. However, activities continued for 5 days in patients with minor leakage. Changes in amylase activities in 12 cases without leakage are shown in Fig. 3. One day after the operation, amylase activities in patients with fibrin sealant were lower than those in the patients without. Two days later, the same result as the day before was observed, thereafter no definite difference could be determined between the two groups.

Incidence of Postoperative Complications

Fortunately, serious pathophysiological conditions were not observed in any of the patients in this study, due to the accurate drainage position. In pancreatoduodenectomy, infections around the anastomosis were found in about 6%–10% of cases (Fig. 4). The incidence of cholangitis or wound infection was lower: 2%–6% (not shown in data). In distal pancreatectomy, the results were very similar to those in pancreatoduodenectomy, the incidence of abdominal infection was slightly higher, whereas the occurrence of cholangitis was not observed (not shown in data). Further, as the latter results indicate, the abso-

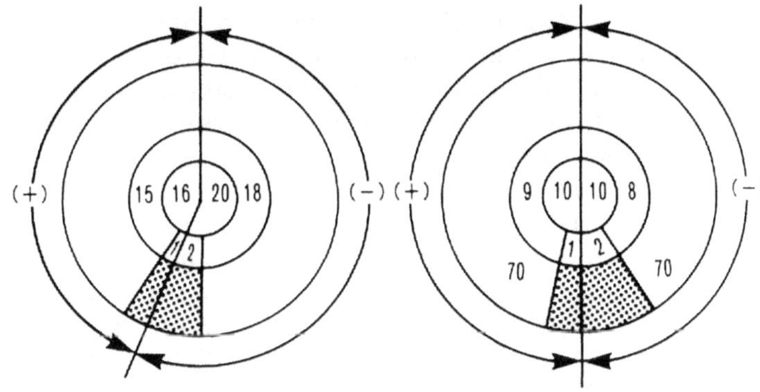

Fig. 4. Incidence of abdominal infections after pancreaticojejunostomy (*left*) and pancreatectomy only (*right*). *Shaded areas* indicate cases with complications. +, Fibrin sealant used; –, fibrin sealant not used

lute number of patients with complications, i.e., intra-abdominal infection and anastomotic insufficiency, was more or less the same because of the simultaneous occurrence.

The occurrence of postoperative local complications in distal pancreatectomy is mainly due to technical causes involving the resected surface of the pancreas. The macroscopical bleeding should principally be arrested by ligation or coagulation, minor bleeding, the pancreatic juice leakage, and fluid secretion in the resected surface might induce infection or abscess, and this cannot be avoided in a few patients, however much care is taken. Of the 36 pancreaticojejunostomies and 20 distal pancreatectomies, the number of cases with minor leakage of pancreatic juice is given in Fig. 5, according to the different treatment, i.e., the usage of fibrin sealant. Absolute numbers of the cases with minor leakage of four in pancreaticojejunostomy and two in distal pancreatectomy. The incidence of minor leakage in the nonusage group is higher than that

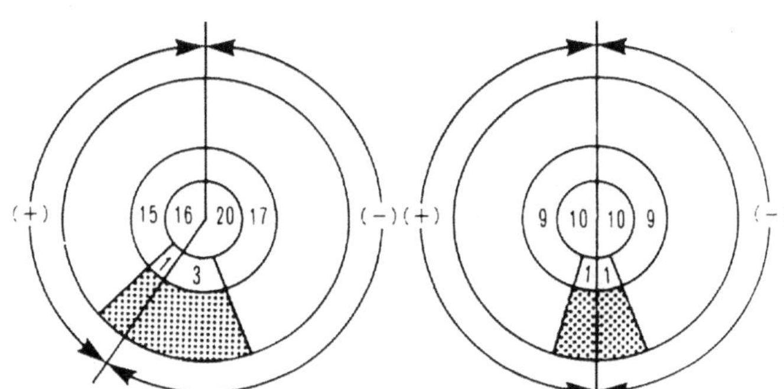

Fig. 5. Incidence of minor leakage of pancreatic juice after pancreaticojejunostomy (*left*) and pancreatectomy only (*right*). *Shaded areas* indicate cases with complications. +, Fibrin sealant used; –, fibrin sealant not used

of the usage group in pancreatoduodenectomy, but no difference between the two groups is found in distal pancreatectomy. The interval between the occurrence of leakage and draining was compared, according to whether or not fibrin sealant was used (Fig. 6). In pancreaticojejunostomy, the interval in patients in which fibrin sealant was used is clearly shorter than in the three cases without. In distal pancreatectomy, the intervals in two cases (one with and one without) showed the same results. In the same way as with the study of minor leakage of pancreatic juice, the incidence of abdominal infections in pancreatoduodenectomy and distal pancreatectomy were studied, according to whether or not fibrin sealant was used. The absolute numbers of patients with abdominal infections are completely accordant with those of the cases with minor leakage, because this complication was mostly caused by the minor leakage. Simple bacterial infections were found in four cases (two *Klebsiella*, one *Staphylococcus*, and one *Pseudomonas*) and compounded bacterial infections were found in two cases (*Klebsiella* plus *Streptococcus* and *Enterobacter* plus *Staphylococcus*). Bacterial infection did not depend on whether fibrin sealant was used.

Discussion

This study reports the incidence of local complications after pancreatic operations and extends the confirmation of the effect of fibrin sealant in protecting against anastomotic insufficiency of pancreaticojejunostomy and against leakage of pancreatic juice from the resected surface of pancreas as well as its effects on hemostasis. Several methods of management to avoid pancreatic fistula have been reported [2, 7]. The method of complete obstruction of the

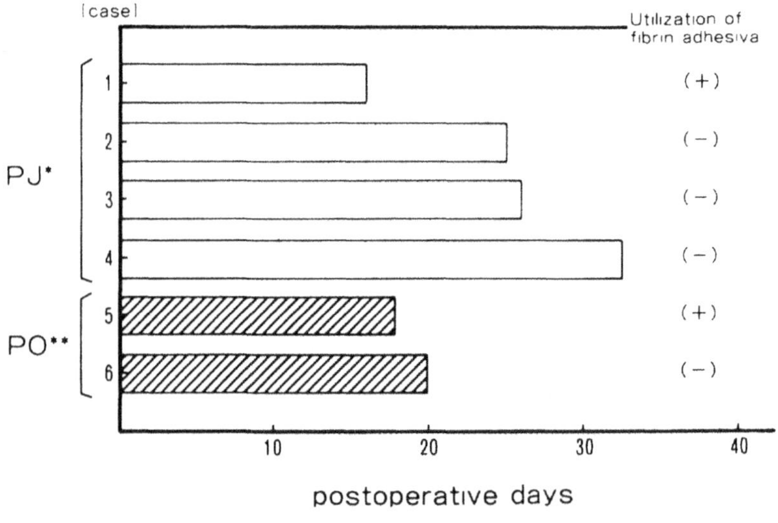

Fig. 6. Drainage interval in cases with minor leakage of pancreatic juice. *White bars*, pancreaticojejunostomy; *shaded bars*, pancreatectomy only

pancreatic duct is well known. However, the maintenance of pancreatic parenchyma was difficult and therefore there were clearly limitations in the preservation of pancreatic function. We have realized that identification of the main pancreatic duct and precise drainage to it are likely to prevent the occurrence of local complications, but it is impossible to completely avoid such complications.

Recently, the beneficial effects of fibrin sealant on the healing process and on hemostasis have become well known in surgical treatment; however, the number of reports comparing early outcome of pancreatojejunostomy with and without fibrin sealant has not been enough. Even the question of whether the formation of a fibrin network in the presence of pancreatic juice is permanent, has not been clarified.

Therefore, it seems likely that most surgeons in the field of gastrointestinal medicine have not utilized fibrin sealant on pancreaticojejunostomy as an additional material. Basic studies have demonstrated disorders of coagulation behavior as one of protein response in various pathophysiologic conditions. Such disorders induce anastomotic insufficiency [1, 9], because of the additional burden caused by extended radical operation of pancreatoduodenal malignancies. Most complications, however, are thought to have resulted from minor technical errors. It is thought that the technical aspect of pancreaticojejunostomy has four important components: (1) the drainage of pancreatic juice from the main pancreatic duct, (2) the suture of the pancreatic parenchyma and intestinal wall, (3) the suture of the pancreatic seroparenchyma and the seromuscular layer of intestine, and (4) hemostasis of the respected surface of the pancreas. Among these technical points, fibrin sealant is realized to be useful, especially for the latter three techniques. In order to confirm the effect of fibrin sealant in these points, it was only applied in the suture of the pancreatic seroparenchyma and the seromuscular layer of the intestine. The results suggest that fibrin sealant is effective in protection against local complications. However, the poor standard of clinical data has made it very difficult to confirm this result. Further, the fact that no difference was found in statistics comparing the two groups (one with fibrin sealant and the other without) might be due to the small number of cases and the lower incidence of complications in this study. Therefore, further studies will be necessary.

In conclusion, it is sure that the occurrence of complications in pancreatic operations was mainly caused by uncomfortable, often ineffective techniques. Fibrin sealant in pancreatoduodenectomy and distal pancreatectomy may be an effective material in preventing pancreatic fistulae and bleeding; however, further investigations are necessary to confirm these preliminary clinical data.

References

1. Ambrus JL, Ambrus CM, Pickern J, Soldes S, Bross I (1975) Hematologic changes and thromboembolic complications in neoplastic disease and their relationship in metastasis. J Med 6: 433–458
2. Fitzgibbons TJ, Yelling AE, Maruyama MM, Donovan AJ (1982) Management of the transected pancreas following distal pancreatectomy. Surg Gynecol Obstet 154: 225–231

3. Kram HB, Clark SR, Ocampo HP, Yamaguchi MA, Shoemaker WC (1991) Fibrin glue sealing of pancreatic injuries, resections, and anastomoses. Am J Surg 161: 379–481
4. Kram HB, Nathan RC, Mackabee JR, Klein SR, Shoemaker WC (1988) Clinical use of nonautologous fibrin glue. Am J Surg 54: 570–573
5. Kram HB, Nathan RC, Stafford FJ, Fleming AW, Shoemaker WC (1989) Fibrin glue achieves hemostasis in patients with coagulation disorders. Arch Surg 124: 385–387
6. Matsuno S, Sato T (1986) Surgical treatment for carcinoma of the pancreas. Experience in 272 patients. Am J Surg 152: 499–502
7. Pachter HL, Pennington R, Chassin J, Spencer FC (1979) Simplified distal pancreatectomy with the autosuture stapler: preliminary clinical observations. Surgery 85: 166–170
8. Papachristou DN, Fortner JG (1981) Pancreatic fistula complicating pancreatectomy for malignant disease. Br J Surg 68: 238–243
9. Sach GH Jr, Levin J, Bell W (1977) Trousseau's syndrome and other manifestations of chronic disseminated coagulopathy in patients with neoplasms: clinical pathophysiologic and therapeutic features. Medicine (Baltimore) 56: 1–37
10. Tashiro S, Murata E, Hiraoka T, Nakamura K, Watanabe E, Miyauchi Y (1987) New technique for pancreaticojejunostomy using a biological adhesive. Br J Surg 74: 392–394

Duct Occlusion with Fibrin Glue After Pancreatoduodenectomy for Periampullary Neoplasms

M. Cavallini and S. Stipa

Abstract

After pancreatoduodenectomy (PD), drainage of a soft pancreatic stump with a narrow duct by pancreaticojejunostomy (PJ) entails the risk of a PJ leakage. Progression to peritonitis and sepsis constitutes a life-threatening situation. Since May 1988, in order to avoid such potentially catastrophic sequelae in 11 patients affected by periampullary neoplasms who were treated with PD and who had a soft pancreatic stump, we have utilized a duct occlusion technique with fibrin glue and without PJ. One further patient was treated with this technique because of his critical respiratory condition in order to shorten the operative time. One patient died (8.3 %) on postoperative day 20 because of sepsis after a relaparotomy for hemoperitoneum caused by gastroduodenal artery bleeding. Nine patients (75 %) had an external pancreatic fistula, which spontaneously healed between 2 weeks and 4 months after surgery and with no other sequelae. At follow-up (3–54 months) all patients were normoglycemic. Two patients already suffering from non-insulin-dependent diabetes (NIDD) before surgery resumed taking oral antidiabetic drugs after hospital discharge.

The aim of using fibrin sealant in these patients was to block pancreatic secretion in the early postoperative period, when intestinal anastomoses are in the process of healing. Although they can create some patient discomfort, the pancreatic fistulae observed have a benign evolution and heal spontaneously in few weeks. The results of this initial experience document that this method of handling exocrine secretion is safe and satisfactory and is, in our opinion, indicated when the pancreas is not sclerotic and leakage of the anastomosis with the jejunum is likely to occur.

Introduction

The surgical approach to pancreatic cancer, one of the deadliest carcinomas in the Western world, has come under scrutiny because of its seemingly limited effect in improving survival. Nevertheless, despite the low rates of curative resections, surgery remains the only opportunity for a cure. Data from recent series [1–3] show that in experienced centers where there is a specific interest in pancreatic surgery, a more favorable outcome can actually be obtained than had previously been described. Surgical options for resection of periampullary neoplasms include pancreatoduodenectomy (PD; Whipple procedure), traditionally considered the treatment of choice for periampullary carcinomas [3], and total pancreatectomy (TP), as advocated by some authors [4].

Dehiscence of pancreaticojejunostomy (PJ) is the main technical postoperative complication after PD [5]. Progression to peritonitis and sepsis constitutes a life-threatening situation. The incidence of this complication is particularly high in cases where the duct is narrow and the pancreatic gland tender. In these cases, to avoid such potentially catastrophic sequelae, some authors favor TP [6], a surgical option considered by many surgeons as an overtreatment which exposes the patient to a diabetes that is difficult to manage. Proposed alternative techniques include direct duct occlusion by absorbable (prolamin) [7] or nonabsorbable (neoprene) [8] polymers or by direct suture [9].

More recently, some authors have utilized fibrin glue, an inert, slowly resorbable substance obtained by mixing thrombin and fibrinogen [10].

In the present report, we describe our experience with direct occlusion of the pancreatic duct with fibrin glue in a consecutive series of patients submitted to PD for periampullary carcinoma and bearing a soft pancreatic stump considered at risk for postoperative early complication of any intestinal anastomosis.

Materials and Methods

From March 1972 until November 1992, a total of 199 patients were evaluated and treated at our unit for periampullary tumors. Tumor resection has been feasible in 109 instances (54 %). Operative technique consisted of six tumorectomies, 75 PD, and 28 total pancreatectomies, with various methods of reconstruction of the intestinal continuity. In particular, intestinal reconstruction after PD was done according to the Whipple-Child procedure in 43 cases (distal gastrectomy with end-to-side gastrojejunostomy) and with a pylorus-preserving technique in 32 cases as described by Traverso and Longmire ([11]; 18 cases) or a modification of this approach with reconstruction through an end-to-end duodenojejunostomy about 15 cm proximally to the end-to-side hepaticojejunostomy ([12]; 14 cases). PJ was performed in 62 patients. In this group of patients, the main postoperative complication was leakage of the PJ, observed in eight cases (13 %). In our experience, this complication carries high related mortality, with five postoperative deaths (62 %). Since May 1988, because of this high rate of complications in cases with a narrow duct and a soft pancreatic gland, considered to be at risk for early complication of any intestinal anastomosis, we preferentially have been using the direct occlusion of the pancreatic duct with fibrin glue and suture [13]. The pancreatic gland was not anastomosed to a jejunal loop. This approach has been utilized in 12 patients (seven males and five females; gender ratio; 1.4:1) with a mean age of 60 years (range, 37–81 years). Primary cancer sites included head of pancreas in ten cases (seven stage I and three stage III according to UICC 1987 classification), ampulla of Vater in one case, and distal bile duct in one case. Histology was consistent with adenocarcinoma in 11 cases and APUD cell carcinoma in one case. Indication for PD with duct occlusion without PJ procedure was a soft pancreatic stump in 11 patients; it was also indicated in a patient with respiratory insufficiency in order to shorten the length of the operation. Before surgery, ten patients were normoglycemic, while two patients were type II diabetic under treatment with oral antidiabetic drugs. One patient had had a total gastrectomy 13 years before, with an omega jejunal loop reconstruction because of a gastric ulcer.

The operative technique consisted of standard PD with preservation of the stomach, pylorus, and 2–3 cm of the duodenum. Care was taken to preserve the vagal innervation and the blood supply to the stomach and pylorus. In particular, the vascular arcade of the lesser curvature was preserved by dividing the right gastric artery at its origin. Caution was also taken to preserve the gastroepiploic vessels along the greater curvature of the stomach, dividing the right gastroepiploic artery at its origin from the pancreaticoduodenal artery. Reconstruction was performed by one layer retrocolic end-to-end duodenojejunostomy about 15 cm proximal to the end-to-side hepatico-jejunostomy (Fig. 1). The cut surface of the pancreatic stump was sutured by interrupted stitches.

One of these sutures was placed with U shape around the duct opening and ready to be tied once the duct was occluded with the fibrin glue. The pancreatic stump duct was then cannulated by means of a silastic cannula as deep as possible into the tail (Fig. 2). To make this maneuver easier, a 6–0 monofilament

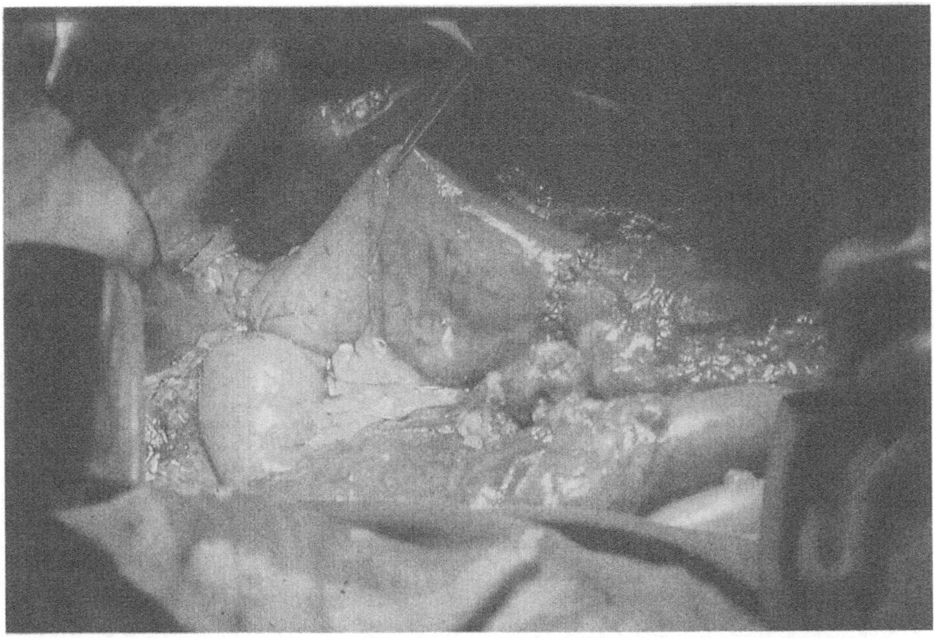

Fig. 1. After pancreatoduodenectomy, intestinal reconstruction is performed with a modification of the pylorus-preserving technique: an end-to-end duodenojejunal anastomosis *(right)* about 15 cm proximal to the hepaticojejunostomy *(left)*

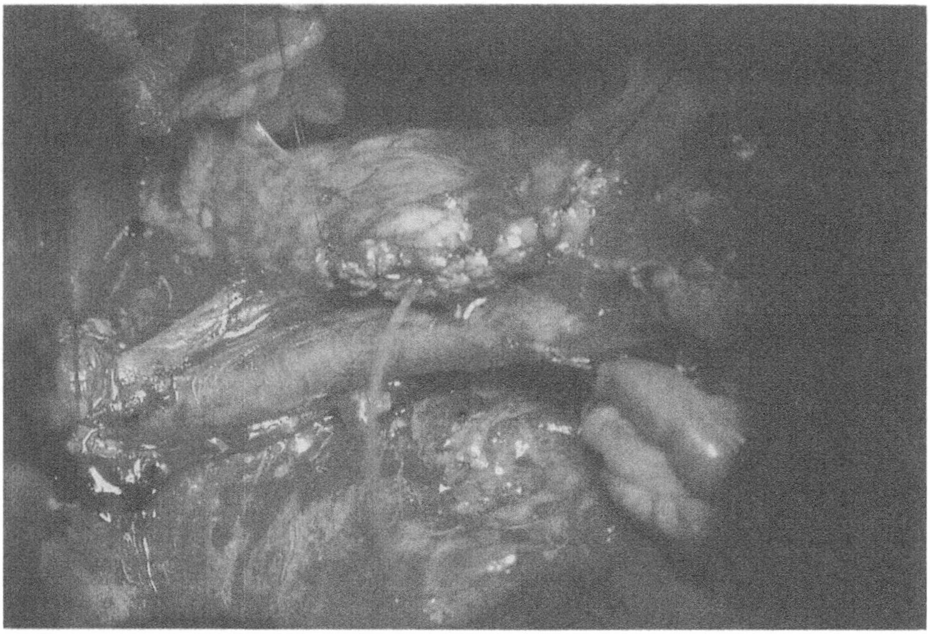

Fig. 2. After pancreatoduodenectomy, the duct of the pancreatic stump is cannulated with a silastic catheter for the fibrin sealant injection

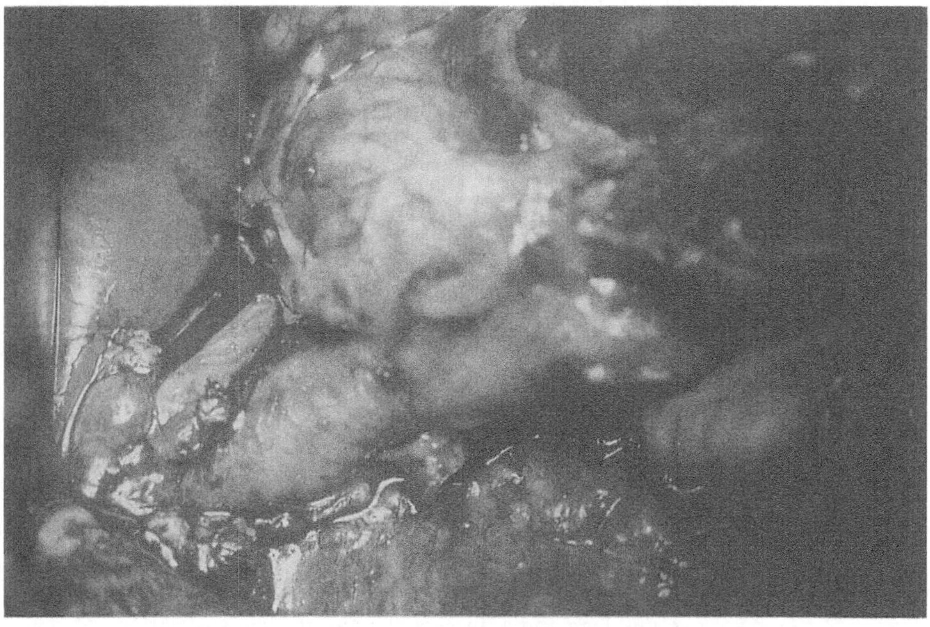

Fig. 3. Fibrin sealant has been injected into the duct and on the cut surface of the gland, while the duct itself has been directly sutured

suture was often placed in the bottom side of the narrow duct and kept steady in order to maintain the opening firm and the duct straight. At this point 3–4 ml fibrin glue was slowly injected while the cannula was removed (Fig. 3). Thereafter, the portion of omentum left was carefully placed behind the stomach (Fig. 4) with the aim of separating the intestinal anastomoses from the area of the pancreatic stump close to the pancreatic gland, where it can participate in the absorption of pancreatic secretion. To complete the operation, two Penrose drains were placed near the pancreas.

Fibrin glue is obtained by mixing two components, thrombin (4 IU/ml) and Tisseel (Immuno, Vienna) diluted with an aprotinin solution of 20 000 kIU/ml, at 37 °C through a special double syringe device; the injection takes no longer than 1 min.

In the postoperative period, all patients received daily somatostatin (4 mg/day for 10 days; seven cases) or octreotide (0.4 mg/day for 10 days; five cases) and antiacid H2-antagonist drugs.

Once oral feeding was allowed, all patients were supplemented with pancreatic enzymes to prevent malabsorption.

At follow-up (range 3--54 months), all survivors were questioned concerning postoperative tachycardia, flushing, nausea, vomiting, early satiety, postprandial cramps, diarrhea, and steatorrhea.

Gastric emptying and pyloric function were evaluated at 3 months from surgery in five patients using radionuclied study with a standard meal consisting of two hard-boiled eggs, 50 g white bread, 250 g canned peaches, and 250 ml milk. One millicurie of Tc-99 m diethilenpentacetic acid (DTPA) was employed as a marker. The gamma emissions were counted at 60 and 90 min over the area identified on the oscilloscope as the stomach. Gastric emptying was expressed at 60 and 90 min as the percentage of residual radioactivity referred to the initial count of the isotope in the stomach after correction for isotope decay. The mean (± SD) of normal values of residual radio-

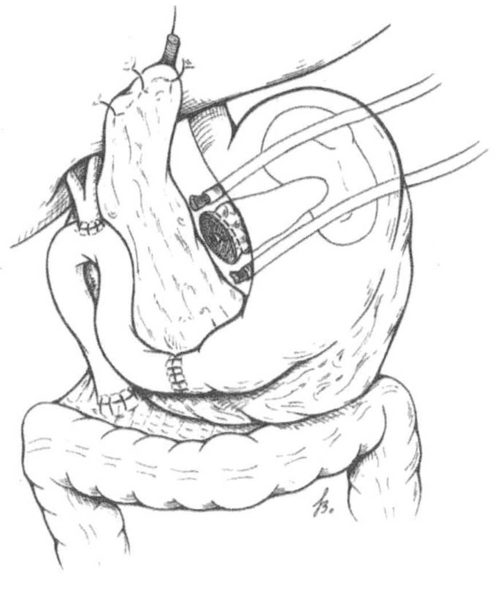

Fig. 4. Pylorus-preserving technique. Note the omentum placed behind the stomach to separate the intestinal anastomoses from the pancreatic stump, which is drained by two Penrose tubes

activity expressed in percentages was obtained in eight healthy volunteers ranging in age from 25 to 45 years: 63.14 ± 6.46% at 60 min and 50.14 ± 4.73% at 90 min.

All patients were evaluated for their fasting blood glucose level, and five patients were evaluated 6 months after surgery for plasma insulin (IRI), glucagon (IRG), and C-peptide (CPR) both under fasting conditions and 1 h after standard meal. Laboratory values in 12 normal subjects (mean ± SE) were 12 ± 3 μU/ml for IRI, 110 ± 22 pg/ml for IRG, and 0.44 ± 0.09 pmol/ml for CPR.

Results

One patient died on postoperative day 20 (8.3%) because of sepsis after an emergency relaparotomy for hemoperitoneum caused by gastroduodenal artery bleeding. The first patient was reoperated on sixth postoperative day to drain a peripancreatic fluid collection. External pancreatic fistula (defined as the collection of amylase-rich fluid) was observed in nine patients (75%). In these patients, the daily drainage volume increased from the second postoperative day on, while the amylase content increased sharply from the third to the fourth postoperative day. Thereafter, the daily volume reached the 400–500 ml level at the end of the first postoperative week. This daily volume then decreased progressively and spontaneously ceased between 2 weeks and 4 months after surgery. In one patient with no postoperative external drainage at 3 months from surgery, a peripancreatic collection of about 350 ml was drained using CT guidance fluid with no further sequelae. Two other patients had external drainage of fluid in the postoperative period, but with a very low concentration of amylases. At follow-up, ultrasound controls were performed periodically every 4–6 months and no other fluid collections were observed after the exhaustion or the progressive reduction of the fistulae.

Of the 11 patients with a pylorus-preserving reconstruction, nine patients had no postoperative complications. Of these latter patients, nasogastric suction was removed after a mean ± SD of 6.6 ± 2.4 days. Gastric emptying studies performed at 3 months after surgery in five patients with a pylorus-preserving technique showed a resumption of gastric function. In this group of patients, mean ± SD residual gastric radioactivity detected at 60 min was 71.5 ± 5.2%, while residual counts recorded at 90 min were 55.6 ± 3.1%. The difference between these values from those observed in the control group (see "Materials and Methods") were not statistically significant. In the early follow-up period, one patient had frequent bowel movements lasting for about 2 months despite pancreatic supplementation. This same patient and another one had occasional abdominal cramps for the first 4 months. None of the patients had steatorrhea, early satiety, tachycardia, flushing, nausea, or vomiting.

All nine normoglycemic survivors had normal fasting serum glucose levels at their follow-up controls or until death occurred. At 6 months after surgery five of these patients had adequate mean hormonal levels both basal and 1 h after a meal: 9.7 ± 4μU (basal) and 35.3 ± 6 μU (after meal) for IRI, 67.2 ±

17 pg/ml (basal) and 65.8 ± 12 pg/ml (after meal) for IRG, and 0.52 ± 0.2 pmol/ml (basal) and 1.4 ± 0.5 pmol/ml (after meal). Two NIDD diabetic patients resumed their oral antidiabetic drugs once discharged from the hospital.

To date five patients have died because of hepatic metastases and cachexy at 3, 9, 10, 14, and 15 months after surgery, respectively. Six patients are alive and apparently disease free at 3, 5, 7, 12, 33, and 54 months after surgery, respectively.

Discussion

In patients affected by periampullary neoplasms and treated by PD, a pylorus-preserving technique appears to be a safe surgical approach [14] also from the point of view of radicality [15]. In the prevention of marginal ulcers after pancreatic surgery, several methods for the reconstruction of the gastrointestinal tract have been proposed, all emphasizing the importance of an extended gastric resection with or without vagotomy and the relevance of bathing the anastomosis itself in biliary and pancreatic juice [16, 17]. However, the pancreatic secretion, which contains the bulk of bicarbonates, is frequently reduced or almost absent after PD because of chronic fibrosis of the residual gland. Moreover, a wide gastric resection cannot always prevent the potential development of anastomotic ulcers. This complication after Whipple operation has been observed in 6%–9% of cases and with vagotomy in 4%–12% of cases [16, 17]. A review of 258 cases of pylorus-preserving technique has documented a 3% incidence of peptic ulcer [14], while in a subsequent study on 87 patients [18], the observed incidence was 6%. In our group of patients, jejunal ulcer was not observed with this technique.

Another complication associated with this procedure is delayed gastric function, which is observed in up to 50% of cases and which generally normalizes in the months following the operation [18], as was the case of our observation.

Therefore, this technique is at least as safe as the Whipple procedure and has some advantages, such as a more physiological reconstruction of intestinal continuity and the preservation of gastric function.

The indication for the use of the duct occlusion technique in this series of patients was the presence, in 11 cases, of a normal, soft gland which is considered to be at risk for early complication of any attempted intestinal anastomosis. In one patient with critical respiratory conditions, this choice was due to the need to reduce the operation time. PJ leakage exposes the patient to peritonitis and sepsis, which constitute a life-threatening situation. In our experience, this complication was observed in eight out of 62 PD (13%). The high incidence of related mortality in this group of patients (five out of eight; 62%) has encouraged us to find an alternative technique for handling pancreatic secretion in that particular condition. It is, in fact, our opinion that in the case of a pancreatic gland site of fibrotic chronic pancreatitis, leakage of the intestinal anastomosis is not likely to occur. The high incidence of pancreatic fistula observed in our patients after duct occlusion technique (75%) can create some patient discomfort, but, on the other hand, these fistulae have a very benign course with a spontaneous resolution within a few weeks of surgery (up to 4 months). This kind of complication is a well-known aspect of pancreas transplantation, and omentoplasty and functioning external drainage are the correct solutions to the problem [19].

The utilization of fibrin glue before direct suture of the duct, in our opinion, is justified by the need to block the pancreatic secretion at least in the first 2–3 days after surgery, when the intestinal anastomoses are in the process of healing. Moreover, the use of a biologically inert, absorbable substance could probably avoid the pancreatic fibrosis induced by nonabsorbable polymers widely employed in experimental and clinical pancreas transplantation [20]. At follow-up, chemical and hormonal controls in our long-term survivors show that the pancreatic stumps maintain adequate homeostasis of carbohydrate metabolism even several months after surgery.

In conclusion, in order to reduce operative mortality and morbidity and to improve the quality of life of malnourished, jaundiced neoplastic patients, we believe that preservation of the stomach can be a useful, more physiological technique after pancreatic resection. When the pancreas is not sclerotic and dehiscence of the anastomosis with the jejunum is likely to occur, it is advisable to occlude the duct with fibrin glue and to leave two Penrose drains in place.

References

1. Trede M, Scwall G, Saeger HD (1990) Survival after pancreatoduodenectomy. Ann Surg 211: 447–458
2. Cameron JL, Crist DW, Sitzmann JV, Hruban RH, Boitnott JK, Seidler AJ, Coleman JA (1991) Factors influencing survival after pancreaticoduodenectomy for pancreatic cancer. Am J Surg 161: 120–125
3. Warshaw AL, Fernandez-del Castillo C (1992) Pancreatic carcinoma. N Engl J Med 326: 455–465
4. Brooks JR, Brooks DC, Levine JD (1989) Total pancreatectomy for ductal cell carcinoma of the pancreas: an update. Ann Surg 209: 405–410
5. Peters JH, Carey LC (1991) Historical review of pancreatoduodenectomy. Am J Surg 161: 219–225
6. Lygidakis NJ, Brummelkamp WH, Tytgat GH, Huibtegtse KH, Lubbers MJ, van der Meer AD, Schenk KE, van Gulik TM, Roesing H (1986) Periampullary and pancreatic head carcinoma: facts and factors influencing mortality, survival and quality of postoperative life. Am J Gastroenterol 81: 968–974
7. Lorenz D, Wolff H, Waclawiczek HW (1988) Die Pancreasgangocclusion in der Resektionbehandlung der chronischen Pankreatitis und des Pankreaskopfcarcinoms. Chirurg 59: 90–95
8. Di Carlo V, Chiesa R, Pontiroli AE, Carlucci M, Staudacher C, Zerbi A, Cristallo M, Braga M (1989) Pancreatoduodenectomy with occlusion of the residual stump by neoprene injection. World J Surg 13: 105–111
9. Papachristou DN, Fortner JG (1981) Pancreatic fistula complicating pancreatectomy for malignant disease. Br J Surg 68: 238–240
10. Waclawiczek HW, Kaindl H (1989) Pancreatic duct occlusion with fibrin sealant for the protection of pancreatic-digestive anastomoses following resection of the pancreatic head. Experimental and clinical study. In: Progress in fibrin sealing. Waclawiczek HW (ed) Springer, Berlin, Heidelberg, New York, pp 79–96

11. Traverso LW, Longmire WP (1980) Preservation of the pylorus in pancreaticoduodenectomy: a follow-up evaluation. Ann Surg 192: 306–310
12. Stipa S, Tersigni R, Cavallini M, Stipa F (1989) Pylorus-preserving total pancreatectomy and segmental pancreas autotransplantation. Ital J Surg Sci 19: 345-354
13. Cavallini M, Tallerini A, Stipa F (1991) Pancreatic duct occlusion with fibrin sealant and pylorus preserving technique after duodenopancreatectomy for periampullary carcinoma. Minerva Chir 46: 733–739
14. Itani KM, Coleman RE, Mayers WC, Akwari OE (1986) Pylorus-preserving pancreatoduodenectomy. A clinical and physiologic appraisal. Ann Surg 204: 655–665
15. Klinkenbijl JHG, van der Schelling GP, Hop WCJ, van Pel R, Bruining HA, Jeekel J (1992) The advantages of pylorus-preserving pancreatoduodenectomy in malignant disease of the pancreas and periampullary region. Ann Surg 216: 142–145
16. Grant CJ, van Heerden JA (1979) Anastomotic ulceration following subtotal and total pancreatectomy. Ann Surg 190: 1–5
17. Rignault D, Halker P, Escourro UJ, Brun JG (1979) Les ulceres anastomotiques après duodenopancreatectomie. Chirurgie 1105: 898–893
18. Braasch JW, Rossi RL, Watkins E JR, Deziel DJ, Winter PF (1986) Pyloric and gastric preserving pancreatic resection. Ann Surg 204: 411–418
19. Dubernanrd MJ, Traeger J, Devonec M, Toutaine JL (1980) Pancreatic transplantation in man: surgical technique and complications. Transplant Proc 12 [Suppl 2]: 40–43
20. Traeger J, Dubernard JM, Touraine JL, Malik MD, Ruitton C (1980) Clinical experience with 15 neoprene-injected pancreatic allografts. Transplant Proc 12 [Suppl 2]: 44–50

Pancreatic Duct Occlusion with Fibrin Sealant for the Protection of the Pancreatic-Digestive Anastomosis Following Resection of the Pancreatic Head (Experimental and Clinical Study)

H. W. WACLAWICZEK and O. BOECKL

Abstract

A dehiscence of the pancreatic-digestive anastomosis occurs even when a healthy lienal pancreas segment, following head resection due to carcinomas, has to be connected with the intestine. The incidence of postoperative anastomotic leaks and pancreatic fistulae is reported to be up to 35 %. A reduction of these postoperative complications has already been achieved by pancreatic duct occlusion (PDO) with prolamin because a quick, irreversible exocrine insufficiency results and the disturbing exocrine secretion is eliminated, but there is still ongoing controversy concerning the possibility of endocrine damage with this method.

Therefore, the goal of our experimental study in domestic pigs ($n = 30$) was to block exocrine secretion only temporarily by PDO with fibrin sealant (FS) in order to ensure safe protection of the anastomosis, but to avoid exocrine and endocrine damage. Our long-term studies up to 6 months postoperatively showed that a high local concentration of aprotinin (fibrinolysis inhibitor) of 20000 IU/ml, added to the FS, is necessary to block exocrine secretion for 5 days postoperatively. Contrary to PDO with prolamin, only moderate interstitial fibrosis of the exocrine tissue remained and no damage of the endocrine function occurred. The pancreatic-digestive anastomoses were healed without complications.

So far this new and effective method for the transient protection of the anastomosis during its most critical period has been employed successfully in 80 patients within the framework of Whipple's operations due to pancreatic head carcinomas. The lethality rate was 1.2 %, the morbidity rate 8.2 %. In the observation period of up to 56 months, exocrine and endocrine insufficiencies occurred only in less than 5 % of cases.

Introduction

The tissue-specific nature of the pancreas parenchyma – especially its tryptic activity – causes a high complication and mortality rate following pancreas resections. The pancreatic-digestive anastomosis is especially at risk when a healthy lienal pancreatic rest has to be connected with the intestine after resections for carcinoma, but it can also be problematic after segmental pancreas transplantations. Therefore, this anastomosis is regarded as the weak point of Whipple's operation (partial pancreatoduodenectomy). In the literature, the incidence of postoperative anastomotic leaks and pancreatic fistulae following pancreaticojejunostomy is reported to be 5%–35%. The average mortality after partial pancreatoduodenectomies is approximately 14% (1.3%–36.3%) [3, 13, 16].

Previously, in order to avoid these complications, many surgeons extended their resection in cases of ductal pancreatic carcinoma and chronic pancreatitis to a total pancreatoduodenectomy. However, the risk of refractory postoperative diabetes had to be accepted. Total pancreatoduodenectomy is at present only a makeshift solution [4].

Advanced surgical techniques and suture materials as well as the growing experience of surgeons due to more frequent indications for partial pancreatoduodenectomies and pancreas transplantations have resulted in the reduction of postoperative complications [6, 14]. In contrast to interventions for chronic pancreatitis, the incidence of anastomotic dehiscences still remains significant in carcinoma and transplantation surgery. The disturbances of the healing process of the pancreatic-digestive anastomosis are caused almost without exception by exocrine pancreas secretion and account for most of the complications.

For this reason, numerous methods for the temporary or permanent elimination of exocrine pancreas secretion have been attempted. The *pancreatic duct ligature method* has fallen out of favor due to its irreversible effects on endocrine function as well as the provocation of acute pancreatitis secondary to accumulation of pancreatic secretion [12].

Attempts at medical control of the exocrine pancreas have been tried using *drugs* such as somatostatin, glucagon, calcitonin, atropin and proteinase inhibitors. Despite promising reports, the lack of proof in eliminating exocrine secretion as well as their high cost make the use of these agents controversial [8].

Drainage of pancreatic juice into the peritoneal cavity without anastomosis leads to pancreatic fistulae or to transitory pancreatogenic ascites, which is absorbed by the peritoneum. Due to high intra-abdominal pressure, pancreatic secretion stops after several weeks, ultimately resulting in duct obliteration and fibrosis [7, 18]. Today this procedure has been abandoned in favor of pancreatic duct occlusion (PDO).

External drainage of pancreatic secretion from the lienal pancreatic segment after partial pancreatoduodenectomy or pancreas transplantation is a method frequently reported. The pancreatic duct is intubated with a thin balloon catheter and the pancreatic secretion is drained through the abdominal wall [15]. However, since carcinoma patients frequently have soft parenchyma and extremely narrow ducts, the use of this procedure is not possible in most cases.

The use of PDO to eliminate exocrine secretion with histoacryl (Braun-Melsungen) was researched experimentally by Little for the first time in 1977 [9]. In 1978, Dubernard used neopren for occlusion in segmental transplantations successfully in experiments and clinically [1]; however, these occlusion agents are nonabsorbable substances.

In 1978, Gebhardt and Stolte applied prolamin to occlude the pancreatic duct in animal experiments. Because of its low viscosity, prolamin can be injected easily, occludes even the smallest pancreatic ductuli, and is phagocytized by leukocytes within 14 days. However, complete atrophy and fibrosis of the exocrine pancreas result and so a total elimination of the exocrine secretion takes place [5]. The severity of the damage caused by this sclerosis on endocrine function remains a point of controversy in the literature [6, 10, 11, 17].

Since 1979, prolamin (Ethibloc) has mainly been used for the occlusion of the lienal pancreas after partial pancreatoduodenectomy for chronic pancreatitis, because this procedure unites two important advantages: prevention of further inflammatory attacks by the quick and complete elimination of exocrine function due to fibrosis and thus an extensive reduction of postoperative complications, especially pancreatic-digestive anastomotic leaks [2].

While little controversy remains after 10 years of clinical experience with prolamin occlusion in chronic pancreatitis, opinions about the use of PDO only of the protection of the anastomosis in carcinoma and transplantation surgery differ greatly. The opponents of prolamin occlusion attribute the improvement of operative results to advanced surgical techniques and thus do not accept the need for loss of exocrine secretion, because concomitant damage to endocrine function cannot be ruled out [6, 10].

For this reason, we have used a new occlusion agent: fibrin sealant (FS). The goals of our studies of PDO with FS were: (a) the short-term blockade of exocrine secretion in the healthy lienal pancreas after pancreatic head resection to protect the pancreatic-digestive anastomosis during healing (approximately 5 days); (b) the prevention of an exocrine atrophy and fibrosis; and (c) avoiding damage to endocrine function.

Materials and Methods

The Occlusion Agent Fibrin Sealant

The principle of fibrin sealing represents the last phase of blood coagulation: highly concentrated fibrinogen solution (factor I) is coagulated with thrombin (factor IIa) and the fibrin stabilizing factor XIII in the presence of calcium ions (factor IV). This results in an insoluble fibrin polymer possessing a high mechanical stability. The speed of clotting is directly dependent on the thrombin concentration. The fibrin clot is dissolved when the fibrinolytic system is activated and the proenzyme plasminogen is transformed into the active protease plasmin. This dissolution is also stimulated by enzymes such as factor XIIa and by proteases such as trypsin. Consequently, especially on tissues with high fibrinolytic activity (such as prostata, lung, and mainly pancreas), it is necessary to add fibrinolytic inhibitors to the sealant in order to protect the fibrin clot against premature dissolution. Aprotinin has proven to be a natural proteinase inhibitor with special effects on trypsin and plasmin.

For the last 15 years, the FS Tissucol (Immuno, Vienna) has been in clinical use. It was applied in all our experiments and clinical cases.

Animal Experiments

We used 2-month-old domestic pigs with an average weight of 20 kg (18–22 kg). The common bile duct and pancreatic duct of domestic pigs have separate orifices in the duodenum, approximately 10 cm apart. Due to this anatomy and the presence of a separate blood supply to the duodenum and pancreas, the duodenum can be preserved during resection of the pancreatic head. All surgical interventions were carried out under endotracheal anesthesia.

Our experiments attempted to answer the following questions: (a) the suitability of FS as an occlusion agent; (b) the concentration of aprotinin required to prevent premature dissolution of FS in pancreatic juice; (c) the optimal time period of PDO required to protect the pancreatic-digestive anastomosis during its healing, while avoiding possible damage to the endocrine function of the pancreas; (d) the specific advantages of PDO with FS versus prolamin; and (e) the identification of possible clinical indications for PDO with FS.

Pancreatic Duct Occlusion of the Lienal Pancreas with Fibrin Sealant

In vitro Experiments with Fibrin Sealant Regarding Its Fibrinolysis in the Pancreatic Juice

In order to investigate the fibrinolysis of FS in vitro, the pancreatic juice of one pig was gathered in five test tubes after stimulation of exocrine secretion with secretin. Into these tubes fibrin clots of 0.5 ml each were added. The thrombin quantity remained constant at 500 IU/ml, while the aprotinin concentrations were 3000, 5000, 10 000, 20 000, and 40 000 IU/ml. The dissolution (fibrinolysis) of these fibrin clots was determined macroscopically at intervals of 6 h.

In vivo Experiments with Fibrin Sealant to Assess Its Elimination from the Pancreatic Duct After Pancreatic Duct Occlusion

Short-term experiments were carried out for 10 days postoperatively. The pancreas of the animals was bisected by a sharp cut above the portal vein.

Group A ($n = 14$). PDO with FS was performed at the pancreatic head via a thin plastic catheter inserted into the duct lumen. FS was applied under pressure using the application set Duploject (Immuno, Vienna). The quantity of thrombin was 500 IU/ml and the aprotinin concentration 10 000 IU/ml. The abdomen was then closed in the standard fashion without drainage.

Group B ($n = 14$). The duct of the lienal pancreas was also occluded with FS, but an aprotinin concentration of 20 000 IU/ml was chosen. Two pigs each underwent relaparotomy on the first, second, third, fourth, fifth, seventh and tenth postoperative days and the following examinations were carried out: (a) macroscopic assessment of duct occlusion of the pancreatic head and tail; (b) stimulation of the exocrine secretion by i.v. injection of secretin and quantitative determination of a possible secretion from the ducts; (c) serum amylase; (d) fasting blood sugar; and (e) after the animals were killed, histological examination of the tissue of the pancreatic head and the lienal pancreas.

Group I: Pancreatic Duct Occlusion of the Lienal Pancreas with Fibrin Sealant After Resection of the Pancreatic Head and Subsequent Anastomosis
Long-term experiments for 6 months postoperatively for the assessment of morphological effects and of exocrine and endocrine functions ($n = 6$). After resection of the pancreatic head and PDO of the lienal pancreas with FS (± 0.7 ml, 500 IU/ml thrombin, 20000 IU/ml aprotinin), anastomosis with the stomach (pancreaticogastrostomy) was carried out and 4 weeks and 6 months later relaparotomies and the following examinations were performed: (a) serum amylase (additionally on the first, fourth, seventh, and 14th postoperative days); (b) i.v. glucose tolerance test (i.v. GTT); (c) basal and glucose-stimulated serum insulin; (d) secretin stimulation test (only after 6 months); (e) macroscopic determination of the anastomosis and the pancreatic tissue; and (f) histological and electron microscopic examinations of the lienal pancreas.

Group II: Pancreatic Duct Occlusion of the Lienal Pancreas with Fibrin Sealant After Resection of the Pancreatic Head and Subsequent Drainage into the Peritoneal Cavity
Long-term experiments for 6 months postoperatively were performed ($n = 6$). The pancreas segments, occluded with FS (± 0.7 ml, 500 IU/ml thrombin, 20000 IU/ml aprotinin), were drained into the peritoneal cavity without anastomosis. The abdomen was closed without drainage. The postoperative examinations were identical to those in group I.

Group III: Pancreatic Duct Occlusion of the Lienal Pancreas with Prolamin After Resection of the Pancreatic Head and Subsequent Anastomosis
Long-term experiments for 6 months postoperatively were performed ($n = 6$). Prolamin (Ethibloc), an alcoholic amino acid solution, was used for PDO of the lienal pancreas following resection of the pancreatic head. A pancreaticogastrostomy was performed as well. The postoperative examinations were identical to those in group I.

Group IV: Anastomosis of the Lienal Pancreas without Pancreatic Duct Occlusion After Resection of the Pancreatic Head
Long-term experiments for 6 months postoperatively were performed ($n = 6$). Following resection of the pancreatic head, only a pancreaticogastrostomy was performed without PDO (examinations identical to those in group I).

Group V: Sham Operations
Long-term experiments for 6 months postoperatively were performed ($n = 6$). After laparotomy only the pancreas was explored.

Clinical Study of Pancreatic Duct Occlusion of the Lienal Pancreas with Fibrin Sealant Following Partial Pancreatoduodenectomies (n = 80)

So far we have used this new method of PDO with FS in 80 cases. These patients (64 men, 16 women) had to undergo partial pancreatoduodenectomies due to papillary or periampullary ($n = 21$) and small ductal ($n = 50$) carcinomas or chronic pancreatitis ($n = 9$). Preoperatively, all patients had normal glucose metabolism.

Surgical technique. After typical partial pancreatoduodenectomy, the pancreatic duct of the lienal pancreas segment was intubated with a thin plastic catheter, through which the FS was applied with the application set Duploject under regular pressure and slow removal of the catheter (Fig. 1).

The average quantity of sealant was 2 (± 0.4) ml. The thrombin and aprotinin concentrations (500 and 20000 IU/ml, respectively) were identical to those in the animal experiments. The occluded lienal pancreas was then anastomosed with the small intestine (single-layer inverting, end to end; Fig. 2).

Postoperative examinations:

- Serum amylase (daily until 12 days postoperatively and after 3 months)
- Fasting blood sugar (daily until the 12th postoperative day, then every 2 months)
- I.v. GTT (after 2 months, 1 year and 2 years)

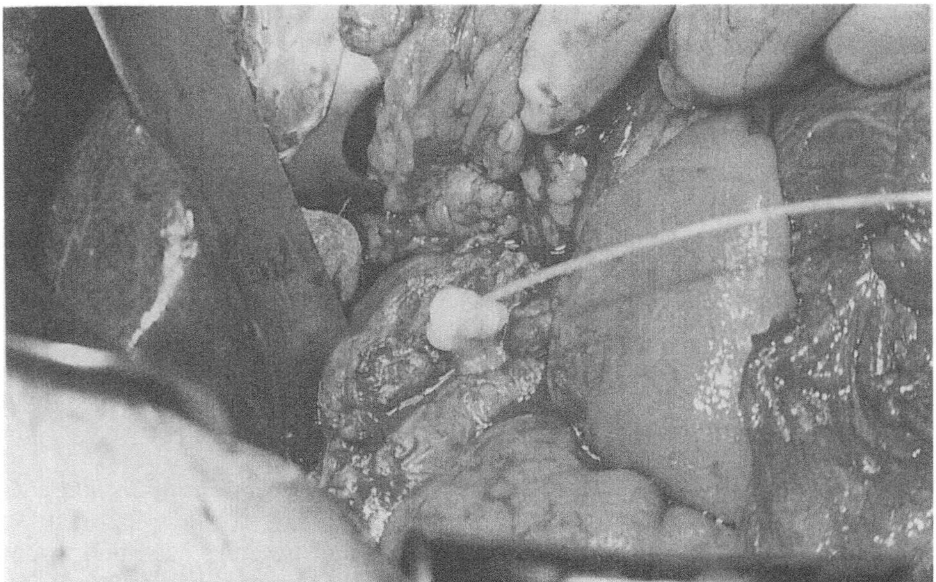

Fig. 1. Pancreatic duct occlusion of the lienal pancreas segment with fibrin sealant following partial duodenopancreatectomy with a thin plastic catheter

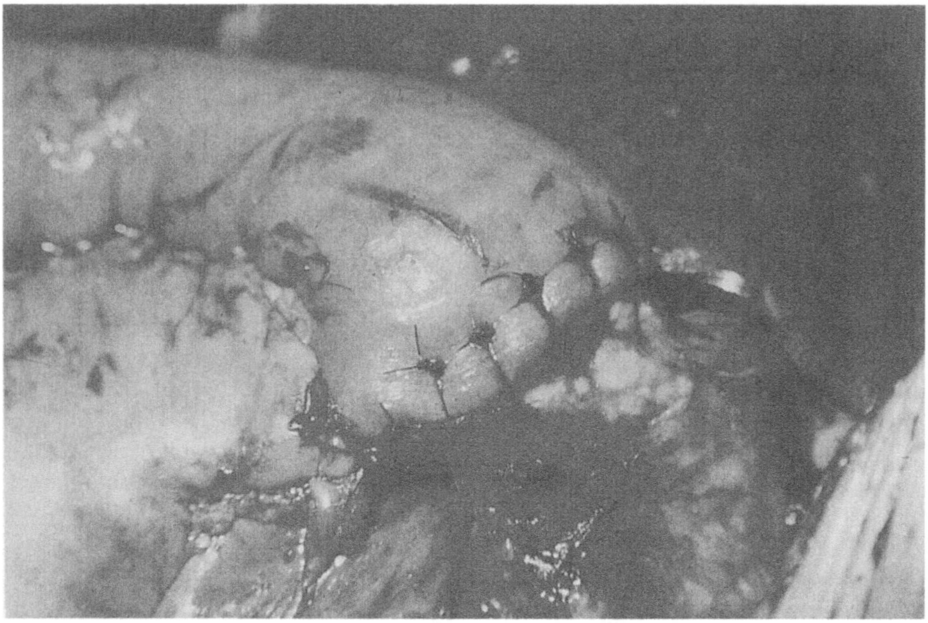

Fig. 2. Pancreaticojejunal anastomosis (single-layer inverting)

Results

Animal Experiments

Pancreatic Duct Occlusion with Fibrin Sealant

In Vitro Experiments with Fibrin Sealant Regarding Its Fibrinolysis in the Pancreatic Juice
The fibrin clot with the usual commercial aprotinin concentration of 3000 IU/ml succumbed to distinct fibrinolysis after 12 h and was completely dissolved after 30 h. The fibrin clots containing 5000 or 10000 IU aprotinin/ml were no longer detectable after 48 and 72 h, respectively. The clot with 20000 IU aprotinin/ml showed the beginnings of fibrinolysis after 60 h and was dissolved on the sixth day. The clot with 40000 IU aprotinin/ml did not succumb to complete fibrinolysis until the eighth day.

Short-Term Experiments of Pancreatic Duct Occlusion with Fibrin Sealant for 10 Days Postoperatively (n = 14)
All animals survived the surgical interventions and two pigs each underwent relaparotomy and were then killed on the first, second, third, fourth, fifth, seventh, and tenth postoperative days, respectively. The serum amylase of all animals rose on the first postoperative day to approximately triple the initial value. After that initial rise, a continual decrease took place until the amylase

normalized after the first week. The PDO caused no significant changes in the fasting blood sugar values.

Group A (10 000 IU Aprotinin/ml.) Macroscopically, the pancreatic duct was occluded with fibrin only in those cases that had undergone relaparotomy before the fourth postoperative day ($n = 6$). The secretion stimulation test showed no evidence of exocrine secretion out of the fibrin-occluded duct up to and including the third postoperative day. From the fourth day on, the quantity of secretion was 16.4 (± 3.2) ml in the 5 min after stimulation (Table 1).

Histologically, the presence of FS in the pancreatic duct could only be seen until the third postoperative day; up to the fifth postoperative day, the interstice was interspersed with edema rich in fibrin. A lymphoplasmohistiocytic pancreatitis existed, but had largely receded by the tenth postoperative day.

Group B (20 000 IU Aprotinin/ml). Macroscopically as well as microscopically, a complete duct occlusion with fibrin existed up to and including the fourth postoperative day. From the fifth postoperative day on, the duct was extensively recanalized. In spite of secretin stimulation no exocrine secretion could be demonstrated until the fourth postoperative day. Thereafter, the quantity of secretion was 15.8 (± 3.5) ml (Table 1).

Also in this trial group, the pancreatic duct could be occluded up to the fifth postoperative day (Fig. 3). The pancreatitis had resolved by the tenth day after PDO.

As a result of these in vitro and in vivo experiments, we used the higher aprotinin concentration of *20 000 IU/ml* in the long-term experiments of PDO with FS (I, II) in order to eliminate exocrine secretion for at least 4 days.

Group I

Serum Amylase. The level rose to 733 (± 76) U/l on the first postoperative day. During the course of the trial, the values decreased rapidly and reached baseline values 2 weeks postoperatively. As compared to groups III (occlusion with prolamin) and IV (sole anastomosis without PDO), there were no significant differences (Fig. 4).

Table 1. Stimulated pancreas secretion up to the tenth day after pancreatic duct occlusion with fibrin sealant (5 min after secretin stimulation)

Postoperative day	Patients	Group A	Group B
	(n)	(ml)	(ml)
1	2	–	–
2	2	–	–
3	2	0.3	–
4	2	10.8 (± 1.5)	–
5	2	16.4 (± 2.9)	11.7 (± 2.2)
7	2	19.7 (± 4.2)	18.3 (± 4.4)
10	2	18.8 (± 4.3)	17.3 (± 4.0)
x		16.4 (± 3.2)	15.8 (± 3.5)

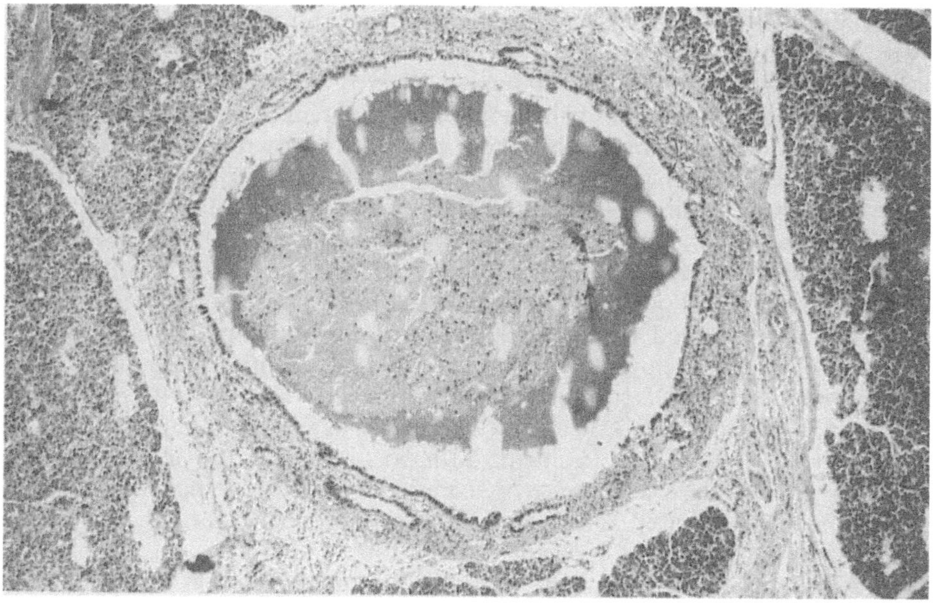

Fig. 3. Complete duct occlusion with fibrin sealant on the fourth postoperative day (group B)

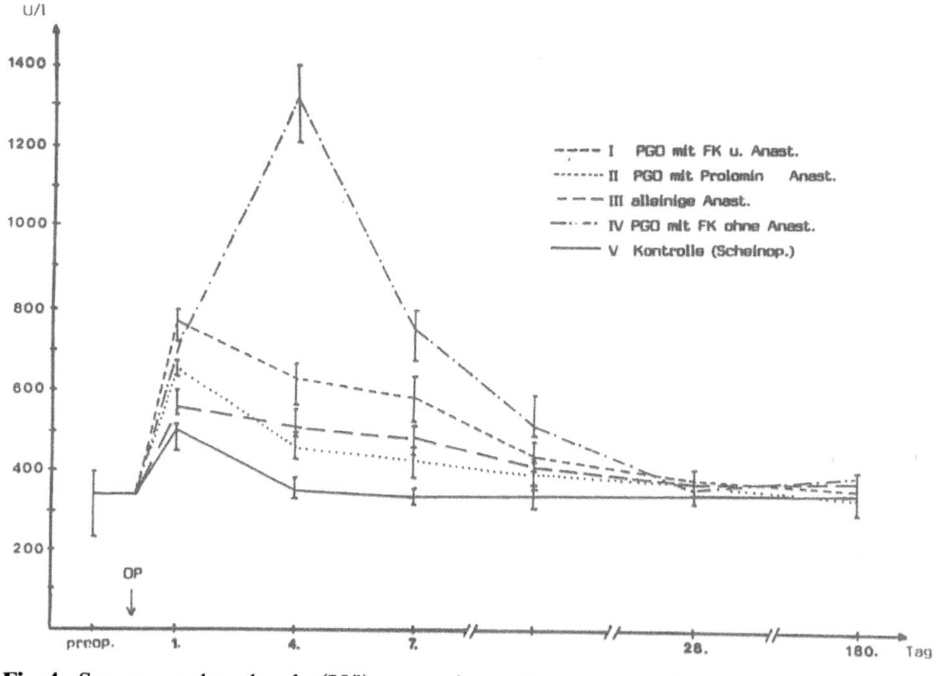

Fig. 4. Serum amylase levels (U/l) up to 6 months postoperatively (groups I–V). See text for details

Exocrine Function. As determined by secretin stimulation tests after 6 months, basal secretion was 1.1 (± 0.6) ml in group I and total secretion was 28.4 (± 11.1) ml in the 10 min after stimulation. In comparison to group IV, there was no significant difference, but compared to groups II, III, and control group V, significantly increased or reduced quantities of secretion were found (Table 2).

Endocrine Function. PDO with FS caused no increase in the fasting blood sugar values compared to the other experimental groups. The analysis of the i.v. GTT also showed no significant differences from preoperative values when compared to the values 4 weeks and 6 months postoperatively (Fig. 5). Compared with the other groups in this trial, no significant differences were found (Fig. 6). The postoperative basal insulin level was 4.2 (± 0.9) μU/l after 4 weeks and 3.9 (± 0.5) μU/l after 6 months and was not significantly reduced when compared with the preoperative values. There were also no significant differences found during both observation periods compared to groups II, III, and IV. After glucose stimulation, no marked deviations of the curves occurred, but the insulin values of all these groups were significantly reduced compared to the control group V (Fig. 7).

Macroscopic Assessment. The anastomoses and pancreatic tissue were assessed macroscopically during the relaparotomies. The pancreaticogastric anastomoses were healed without complications 4 weeks and 6 months postoperatively, and none of the animals showed evidence of acute pancreatitis. The pancreatic ducts were recanalized and were intubated with a catheter far into the pancreatic tail. In all animals, the pancreatic tissue was of soft consistency and macroscopically without pathological findings in both observation periods.

Histological and Electron Microscopic Examinations. Four weeks after temporary PDO with FS these revealed a lymphoplasmohistiocytic interstitial pancreatitis. The larger excretory ducts were moderately dilated and no fibrin could be demonstrated in the ducts. After 6 months the inflammatory changes had decreased with only a moderate interstitial fibrosis remaining (Fig. 8). Normal cytoplasmic granulas of the beta cells could be demonstrated immunohistochemically 6 months postoperatively (Fig. 9).

Table 2. Basal and secretin-stimulated pancreas secretion 6 months postoperatively (groups I–V)

	I (n = 5)	II (n = 5)	III (n = 5)	IV (n = 5)	V (n = 6)
Basal secretion (ml)	1.1 (± 0.6)	0.4	0.2	1.3 (± 0.5)	2.8 (± 0.5)
10 min after secretin stimulation (ml)	28.4 (± 11.1)	2.1 (± 0.7)	1.3 (± 0.7)	33.1 (± 13.9)	62.9 (± 23.3)

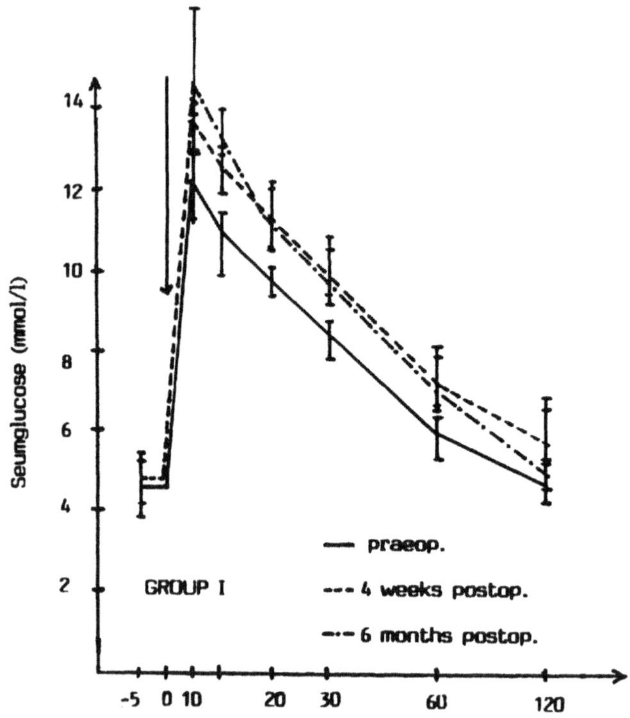

Fig. 5. Intravenous glucose tolerance (mmol/l) up to 6 months postoperatively (group I)

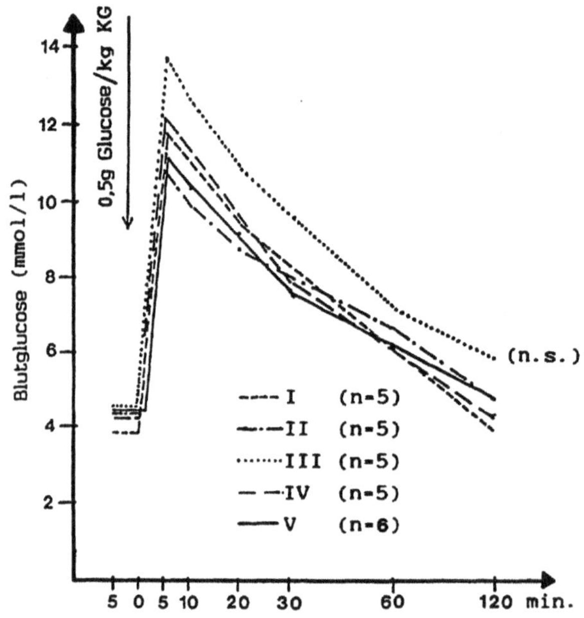

Fig. 6. Intravenous glucose tolerance (mmol/l), 6 months postoperatively (groups I–V). *n. s.*, not significant

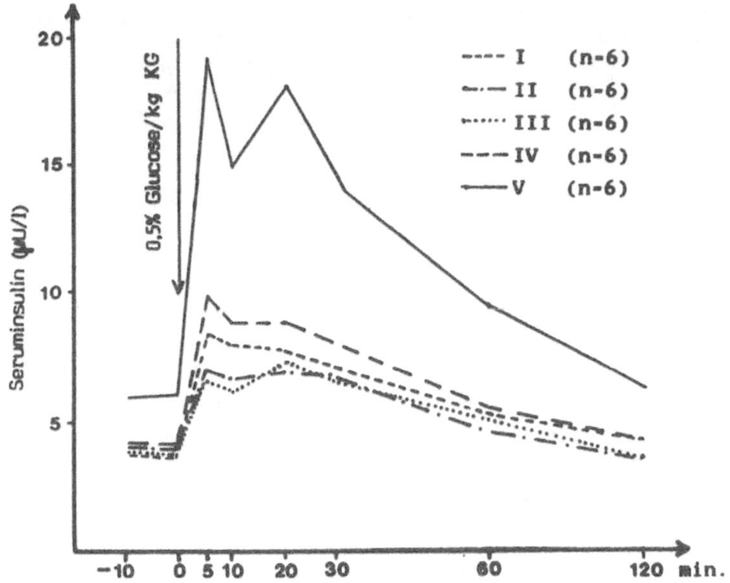

Fig. 7. Basal and glucose-stimulated serum insulin (μU/l), 6 months postoperatively (groups I–V)

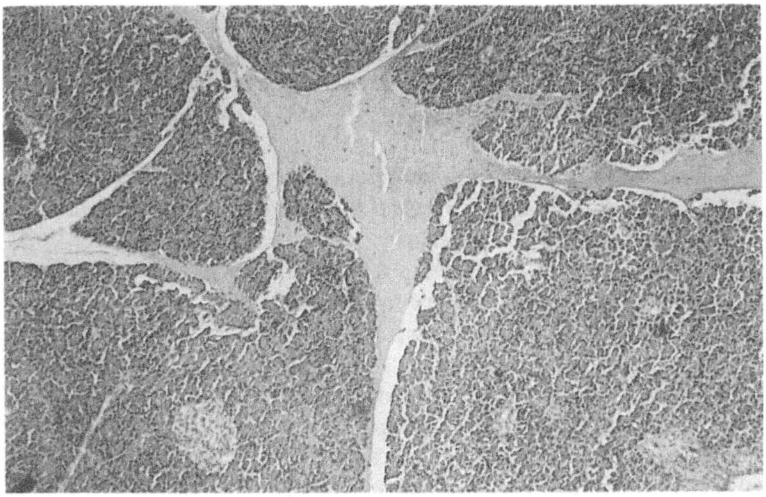

Fig. 8. Soft interstitial fibrosis, 6 months after pancreatic duct occlusion with fibrin sealant (group I)

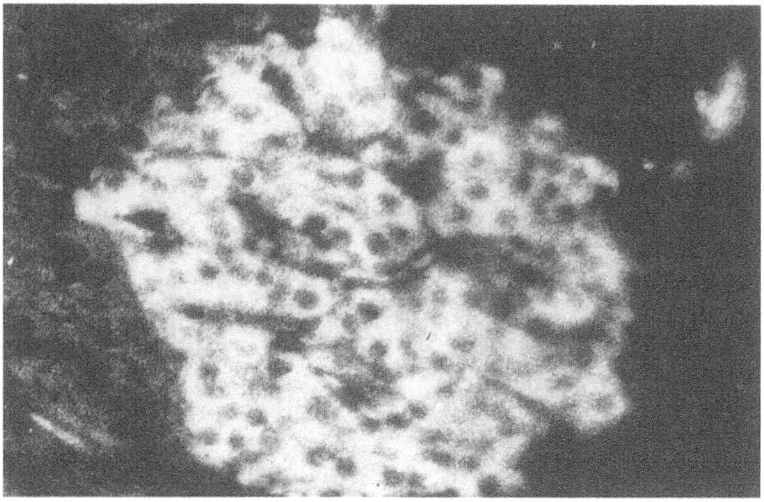

Fig. 9. Immunohistochemical insulin proof, 6 months after pancreatic duct occlusion with fibrin sealant (group I)

Group II

Serum Amylase. The level rose postoperatively up to the fourth day to 936 (± 133) U/l and was significantly increased in comparison to all other groups, but after the third postoperative week the values returned to normal (Fig. 4).

Exocrine Function. Four weeks as well as 6 months postoperatively, basal pancreatic secretion and secretion after secretin stimulation were significantly reduced compared with groups I, IV, and V and approximately corresponded to those of group III (Table 2).

Endocrine Function. The fasting blood sugar values were comparable to normal standards during the first 4 postoperative weeks, but increased slightly after 6 months (not statistically significant). Six months postoperatively, the curves of the i.v. GTT showed a significant increase after glucose stimulation, but were within normal limits at 120 min. As compared to the other groups, the glucose tolerance was not significantly decreases even after 6 months (Fig. 6). Basal as well as glucose-stimulated insulin values showed no marked changes compared to the other groups during both observation periods, but showed a significant reduction when compared to the control group (V; Fig. 7).

Macroscopic Assessment. One of the animals died due to a pancreatic abscess on the 23rd postoperative day. In all other animals a variety of macroscopic changes, ranging from unchanged soft pancreatic tissue to extensive fibrosis, were found 4 weeks and 6 months postoperatively. There were always peripancreatic necroses and moderate pancreatogenic ascites, but the duct lumina were open and easily intubated.

Histological and Electron Microscopic Examinations. In most cases after 4 weeks these revealed chronic interstitial inflammation with collagenous fibers and papillary epithelial proliferations in the excretory ducts, but many Langerhans cells were also seen. After 6 months, the dilatation and induration of the excretory ducts had significantly increased and the exocrine tissue was mostly replaced by connective tissue. However, immunohistochemical examinations at 6 months demonstrated numerous larger Langerhans cells.

Pancreatic Duct Occlusion with Prolamin (Group III)

Serum Amylase. The postoperative level showed a similar course to that of group I during the whole observation time (Fig. 4).

Exocrine Function. In only two of the six animals could a minimal exocrine function be proven 6 months postoperatively (Table 2).

Endocrine Function. PDO with prolamin caused no significant changes of the fasting blood sugar values when compared with the groups occluded with fibrin (I, II) and group IV. In the analysis of the i.v. GTT, the blood sugar values after glucose stimulation increased 6 months postoperatively, but were not significant. Also in comparison to other groups (I, II, IV), no essential deviations resulted (Fig. 6). In the same way, basal and glucose-stimulated serum insulin showed no significant differences to the other groups in both periods (Fig. 7).

Macroscopic Assessment. Anastomoses were assessed during relaparotomy and no leaks, pancreatic fistulae, or pancreatitis were noted. The ducts were dilated up to 6 mm with thickened walls and in all cases the pancreatic tissue was indurated by fibrosis after only 4 weeks.

Histological and Electron Microscopic Findings. After 4 weeks in some cases a massive accumulation of prolamin was found in the dilated excretory ducts. The exocrine pancreatic tissue was already atrophic (Fig. 10). Six months postoperatively, a scarred, indurated inflammation of the interstice with distinct fibrosis and obstruction of the smaller excretory ducts occurred. The Langerhans cells were split up by collagenous tissue, but in all cases the presence of insulin and glucagon was proven by immunohistochemical analyses (Fig. 11).

Anastomosis Only (Group IV)

Serum Amylase. There was a significantly reduced rise in the serum amylase level in this group as compared to groups I, II, and III. After 10 days the values returned to normal (Fig. 4).

Exocrine Function. Basal as well as secretin-stimulated pancreatic secretions were comparable to those of group I, occluded with fibrin (Table 2).

Endocrine Function. Endocrinologically, the fasting blood sugar as well as the i.v. GTT values showed no significant deviations when compared to the other groups (Figs. 6, 7).

Macroscopic Assessment. At relaparotomy 4 weeks later, one case of pancreatic fistula with concomitant peritonitis was found. The animal died due to this anastomotic insufficiency. All the other anastomoses were without pathological findings, and 6 months postoperatively the lumina of the ducts were open.

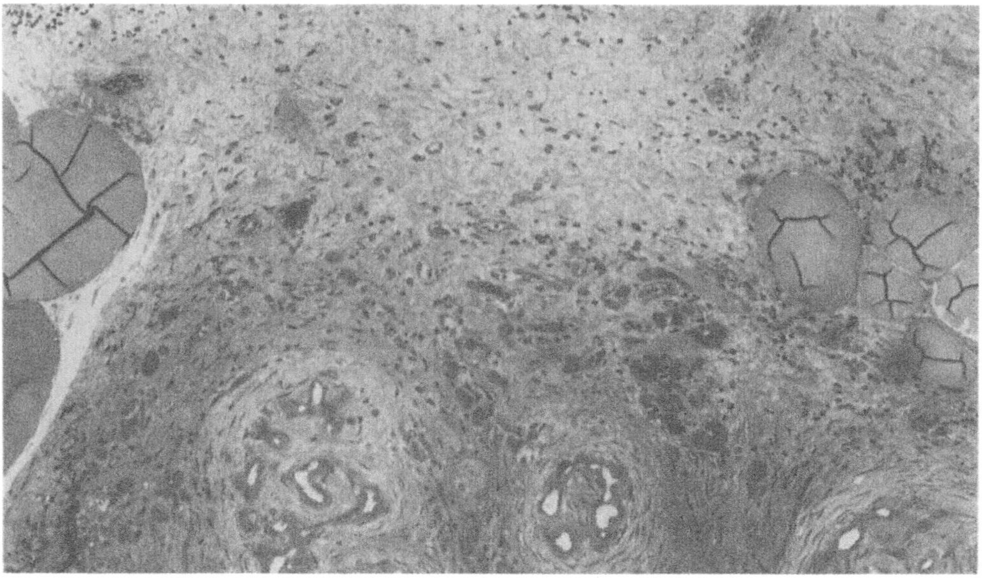

Fig. 10. Extensive atrophy and fibrosis of the exocrine pancreas after pancreatic duct occlusion with prolamin (group III)

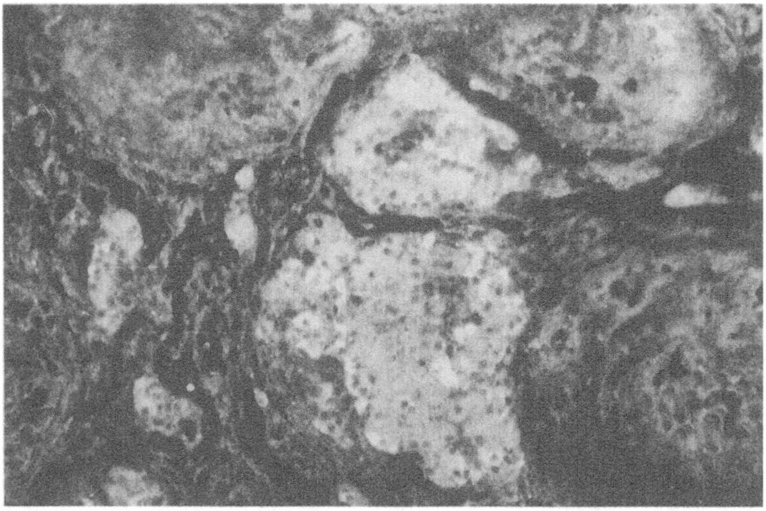

Fig. 11. Langerhans cells split by collagenous tissue (group III)

Histological and Electron Microscopic Examinations. At 4 weeks postoperatively, a lymphoplasmohistiocytic interstitial pancreatitis was found. After 6 months, this fibrosis had progressed only minimally. The grade of this fibrosis was equivalent to that of the fibrin-occluded group I. The presence of large Langerhans cells was proven immunohistochemically.

Clinical Study

A total of 80 patients underwent partial duodenopancreatectomy due to carcinomas ($n = 71$) or chronic pancreatitis ($n = 9$). One patient (78 years old) died on the 21st postoperative day due to cardiorespiratory insufficiency; on autopsy no surgical complication was found. The lethality rate was therefore 1.2%.

Surgical complications occurred in nine cases: biliary fistulae ($n = 3$), partial liver necrosis ($n = 1$), partial colon necrosis ($n = 1$), subcutaneous disturbances of wound healing ($n = 3$), and stenosis of the gastrojejunostomy ($n = 1$). Five of these patients required relaparotomy and further surgical interventions.

No pancreatic fistulae were found. The patients left the hospital after an average of 16 days.

Postoperatively, the serum amylase level rose to triple that of the initial values, but returned to normal within 8 days at the latest. In the observation period (up to 38 months postoperatively) impaired endocrine function was found in only three cases (3.8%), and these patients required insulin. In an additional three cases, severe exocrine insufficiency had to be treated with enzymes.

Discussion

Morphological and Functional Effects of Pancreatic Duct Occlusion with Fibrin Sealant

All experiments were performed with pathologically unchanged organs and thus closely approximated the clinical setting of a pancreas segment after resection due to carcinoma and in segmental pancreas transplantation.

The postoperative serum amylase level after PDO with FS and anastomosis (group I) was comparable to that of group III (occluded with prolamin) regarding the tendency to normalize in the postoperative course. Only after PDO with FS, but without anastomosis (group III), did the serum amylase level rise to triple that of the initial values up to the fourth postoperative day, but thereafter returned to normal.

The drainage of pancreatic secretion into the peritoneal cavity always resulted in a transitory pancreatogenic ascites, which was gradually absorbed by the peritoneum [7].

In groups I (PDO with FS) and IV (anastomosis only without PDO) exocrine pancreatic secretion was reduced by almost half after 6 months in comparison to the control group (V), but this fact may be attributed solely to the reduction of cell mass after resection of the pancreatic head. In the animals occluded with prolamin (group III), no secretion could be demonstrated 6 months later, even after secretion stimulation.

In the long-term experiments, the comparison of endocrine function with a follow-up period of 6 months was of special interest: none of the animals developed diabetes. During the observation periods, the fasting blood sugar, the i.v. GTT, and basal serum insulin showed no significant deviations compared to those of the control animals. Only the values of the glucose stimulated serum insulin were significantly reduced in all occluded groups (I–III), but also in the nonoccluded one (group IV), even 4 weeks after surgical intervention. This too may be accounted for by the quantitative numerical reduction of endocrine cells. These results concur with those of Stolte, who performed electron microscopic examinations of Langerhans cells after PDO with prolamin; a distinct reduction of island cell mass was found [17].

With regard to the morphological effects of PDO, in all groups an identical picture emerged in comparison to the results of the exocrine and endocrine examinations.

In the short-term experiments of PDO with FS, we were able to prove that no grave consequences for the exocrine and endocrine tissue were caused by fibrin occlusion of up to 5 days. After a short period of edema with accompanying pancreatitis, a "mild" interstitial fibrosis resulted, without significant loss of exocrine and endocrine functions. In the long-term experiments of PDO with FS and anastomosis (group I), a reduction of inflammatory changes took place after the fourth postoperative week and resulted in a moderate scarring tendency of the interstice, yet the exocrine tissue was preserved. The grade of fibrosis corresponded with that of the nonoccluded group (IV). Intact endocrine function was demonstrated even 6 months postoperatively by immunohistochemical and glucagon examinations. In comparison, complete atrophy of the exocrine tissue occurred in the group occluded with prolamin (III), a finding consistently reported by others [2, 3, 5]. PDO with FS and drainage into the peritoneal cavity (group II) also resulted in fibrosis with distinct exocrine insufficiency after 6 months. In these two groups, the Langerhans cells were integrated in the scar tissue and partly split up, but endocrine function was only minimally damaged.

Protection of the Anastomosis

Especially in partial pancreatoduodenectomies for carcinoma, but also in segmental pancreas transplantations, the pancreatic-digestive anastomoses are highly endangered because of the tryptic activity of the healthy lienal pancreas. Disturbances of the healing process of the anastomoses are caused mainly by exocrine secretion.

The mere use of additive FS in sutured anastomoses could achieve a reduction in postoperative complications and mortality [19].

PDO with FS provides an additionally high degree of security for the anastomosis. Our comparative study of the different occlusion procedures and of those without PDO admittedly resulted in no significant difference regarding anastomotic dehiscences, but only one animal of the nonoccluded group (IV) died due to complications of anastomotic insufficiency.

Our experiences allow some conclusions to be made regarding the problem of the protection of the anastomosis:

1. Exocrine pancreatic secretion is eliminated for at least 4 days by PDO with FS containing an adequate concentration of aprotinin, allowing the healing of the anastomosis to proceed undamaged.
2. After recanalization of the duct, exocrine function is again intact. While permanent PDO with prolamin also provides an efficient protection of the anastomosis, the complete loss of exocrine secretion must be accepted.
3. During the observation periods of 6 months in the experimental groups and of 38 months in the clinical study, no damage of endocrine functions occurred.

Thus, PDO with FS is a simple and efficient procedure for the transient protection of the pancreatic-digestive anastomosis during its most critical period, and for this reason it can be recommended for partial pancreatic resections in carcinoma surgery as well as in segmental pancreas transplantation. However, fibrin occlusion cannot replace the anastomosis and does not compensate for technical errors.

References

1. Dubernard JM, Traeger J, Neyra P et al. (1978) A new method of preparation of segmental pancreatic grafts for transplantation: trials in dog and men. Surgery 84: 633
2. Gall FP, Zirngibl H (1987) Chirurgie des duktalen Karzinoms. In: Gall FP, Gebhardt Ch. Groitl H (eds) Fortschritte in der Pankreaschirurgie. Zuckschwerdt, Munich
3. Gebhardt C (1984) Akute Pankreatitis. In: Gebhardt C (ed) Chirurgie des exokrinen Pankreas. Thieme, Stuttgart, p 20
4. Gebhardt C, Gall FP, Muehe E, Lauterwald A (1979) Ist die totale Pankreatektomie zur Behandlung der chronischen Pankreatitis noch zu verantworten? Langenbecks Arch Chir 350: 129
5. Gebhardt C, Stolte M (1978) Pankreasgang-Okklusion durch Injektion einer schnell härtenden Aminosäurenlösung. Langenbecks Arch Chir 346: 149
6. Horn J (1985) Anastomosentechniken. In: Horn J (ed) Therapie der chronischen Pankreatitis. Springer, Berlin Heidelberg New York
7. Kyriakides GK, Sutherland DER, Olson I, Miller J, Najarian JS (1979) Segmental pancreatic transplantation in dogs. Transplant Proc 11: 216
8. Landgraf R (1983) Mechanical and hormonal blockade of the pancreatic transplant function in men. Segmental pancreatic transplantation. Thieme, Stuttgart
9. Little JM, Lauer C, Hoog J (1977) Pancreatic duct obstruction with an acrylate glue: a new method for producing pancreatic exocrine atrophy. Surgery 81: 243
10. Lorenz D, Lippert H, Wolff H (1987) Frühergebnisse nach Whipple'scher Operation mit und ohne Gangokklusion. In: Gall FP, Gebhardt C, Groitl H (eds) Fortschritte in der Pankreaschirurgie. Zuckschwerdt, Munich
11. Lorenz D, Wolff H, Waclawiczek HW (1988) Die Pankreasgangokklusion in der Resektionsbehandlung der chronischen Pankreatitis und des Pankreaskopfcarcinomas. Eine 3jährige Nachbeobachtungsstudie. Chirurg 59: 90

12. Martin L, Conseco JD (1947) Pancreatic calculosis. JAMA 135: 1055
13. Meister R (1987) Whipple'sche Operation und Gangokklusion. In: Gall FP, Gebhardt C, Groitl H (eds) Fortschritte in der Pankreaschirurgie. Zuckschwerdt, Munich
14. Sápy P, Mikò I, Furka I (1982) Comparison of suture materials in the pancreas. Acta Chir Acad Sci Hung 23: 209
15. Schopohl J, Zöckler CE, Draese K (1986) Ein modifiziertes Whipple'sches Operationsverfahren. Chirurg 57: 517
16. Sellner f, Jelinek R (1979) Behandlungsergebnisse nach partieller Duodenopankreatektomie. Wien Med Wochenschr 23: 682
17. Stolte M, Lauer E, Bürner W, Zirngibl H, Gebhardt Ch (1987) Elektronenmikroskopische Befunde an den Langerhans-Inseln nach Pankreasgangokklusion. In: Gall FP, Gebhardt Ch, Groitl H (eds) Fortschritte in der Pankreaschirurgie. Zuckschwerdt, Munich
18. Sutherland DER, Goetz FC, Najarian JS (1979) Intraperitoneal transplantation of immediately vascularized segmental pancreatic grafts without duct ligation: a clinical trial. 5th meeting of the American Society of Transplant Surgeons, Chicago, June 1979
19. Waclawiczek HW, Boeckl O (1988) Die Wertigkeit der additiven Anastomosen- bzw. Nahtversiegelung mit Fibrinkleber am Gastrointestinaltrakt. Aktuel Chir 23: 17

Kidney Transplantation from Living Donors with Multiple Renal Arteries, Experiences with Fibrin Sealing

D. Alfani, P. Berloco M. Caricato, R. Pretagostini, F. Carboni, M. Rossi, P. Bruzzone, and R. Cortesini

Abstract

Despite many efforts to increase organ procurement, the persistent shortage of cadaveric kidneys is one of the factors that justifies the use of living donors. New immunosuppressive protocols together with the refinement of surgical techniques now allow us to use living donors such as unrelated donors, older donors, or subjects with bilateral multiple renal arteries, all of whom would have been unsuitable as donors in the past.

From January 1986 until April 1992, among the 322 subjects evaluated for living donation 237 have been accepted, 54 with two and 12 with three renal arteries. In all these cases, multiple renal arteries have been anastomosed on hypothermic bench surgery procedure by 7–0 monofilament running suture to a Teflon (polytetrafluoroethylene) patch. Around the vascular anastomosis between patch and renal arteries, fibrin sealing (Tissucol, Immuno, Vienna) was employed. The patch was then anastomosed to the iliac artery by a running 5–0 suture. The same technique has been employed in one case of renal artery aneurysm at its bifurcation, one case of fibromuscular dysplasia of the renal artery, three cases of adult living kidney donors for pediatric recipients, two cases of older cadaveric kidney donor with bilateral ostial arthrosclerotic lesions, and three cases of unrecognized damaged polar arteries during kidney harvesting.

Homogeneous kidney revascularization followed by immediate urine output was always observed. No surgical complications occurred. Moreover, the comparative prospective analysis with a control group of kidney-grafted patients from living donors with a single renal artery did not demonstrate any difference between the two groups in terms of renal function and blood pressure at 1 and 3 years follow-up.

This technique, with safe and reliable results, enables us to substantially increase the pool of living kidney donors without affecting the long-term results. In fact, the procedure allows the reduction of secondary warm ischemia and homogeneous and simultaneous revascularization of the graft. Furthermore, the use of fibrin sealing helps the confection of the anastomosis using a large growth factor, while reducing the risk of early stenosis or late thrombosis after transplantation. Finally, the use of fibrin sealing does not represent an immunological risk.

Introduction

Renal transplantation is presently considered the most appropriate therapy for end-stage kidney disease. The refinements of surgical techniques have made it possible to harvest organs from donors over 60 years of age or from living donors with multiple renal arteries. Moreover, the shortage of cadaveric donors and the better results obtained after kidney transplantation from living donors have increased the indications for this procedure, which should be performed whenever possible [1].

Here we describe the surgical technique developed by our group for living kidney donors with bilateral anatomical anomalies of the renal artery, which until recently were considered a contraindication to renal transplantation.

Material and Methods

Since 1966, 867 kidney transplantations have been performed at our institutes. The introduction of cyclosporine in 1982 has improved the long-term results and subsequently increased the number of transplant operations [2] (Fig. 1). Before 1985, we evaluated 188 potential kidney donors and excluded 55 of them, in 15 cases as a consequence of bilateral multiple renal arteries. From January 1986 to April 1992, 330 living donors were selected (Table 1), 69 with double and 12 with triple renal arteries. "Triple therapy" using cyclosporine, azathioprine, and low-dose steroids has been used for immunosuppression in all transplant recipients according to the protocols elsewhere described [3].

Donor nephrectomy was always performed without dissecting the vascular structures within the hilus, and the kidney was perfused, immediately after its removal, with EuroCollins at 4 °C. In 70 cases (Table 2) multiple renal ar-

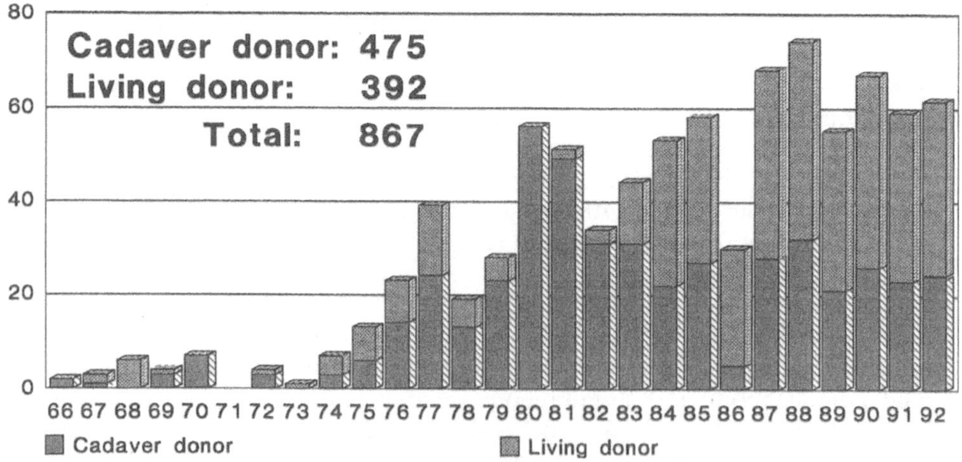

Fig. 1. Overall experience in kidney transplantation at the University of Rome "La Sapienza"

Table 1. Kidney transplantation in the cyclosporine era: experience with 330 kidney transplants from living donors

Donor	Cases ($n = 330$)
Related	223
Unrelated	107
Age > 60 years	21
Multiple renal arteries	81

teries were separately end-to-side anastomosed during hypothermic bench surgery [4] to a Teflon (polytetrafluoroethylene) patch by 7–0 polypropylene continuous sutures (Fig. 2), with a large growth factor; they were subsequently sprayed using a Duploject (Immuno, Vienna) device [5] with fibrin glue (Tissucol, Immuno, Vienna) and rapidly solidifying thrombin (500 IU/ml). The same technique was used in transplantations from a living donor to a pediatric recipient of less than 15 kg, elderly cadaveric kidney donors with ostial atherosclerotic lesions, donor renal artery diseases, recipient vascular pathology, or donor arterial damage during harvesting procedure.

During the transplant operation, the Teflon patch was end-to-side sutured to the recipient's external iliac artery and the renal vein to the external iliac vein by 5–0 polypropylene continuous sutures; a Lich-Gregoire ureterocystoneostomy completed the operation [6].

The follow-up study of the grafted kidneys (range 1–72 months; mean, 30 months) was performed at 3-month intervals by means of biochemical tests, fine needle aspiration biopsy, color Doppler flow mapping, angioscintigraphy, and digital angiography. Moreover, a prospective comparative analysis was performed using a control group of patients who underwent kidney transplantation from living donors with a single renal artery.

Table 2. Kidney transplantation from living donors: surgical techniques of arterial reconstruction in multiple renal arteries

Surgical technique	Cases (n)
Hypogastric bifurcation	9
Epigastric artery	2
Teflon patch	70
Total	81

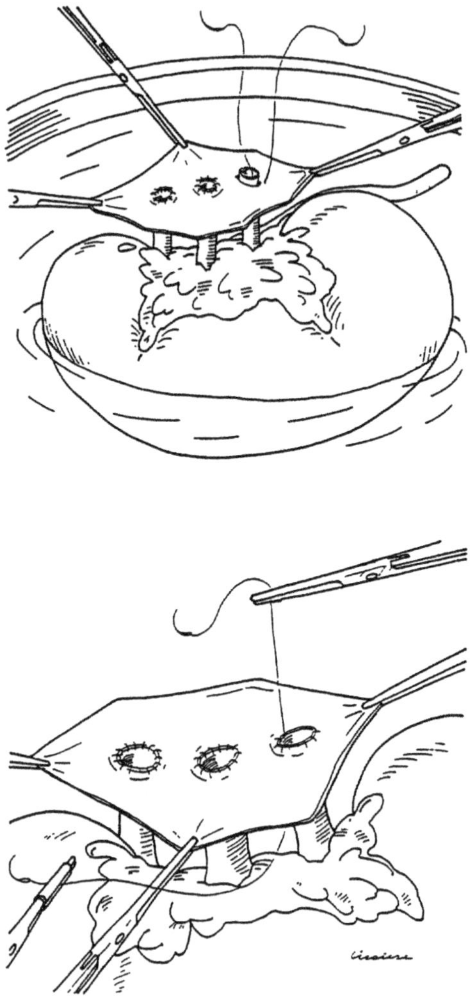

Fig. 2. End-to-side anastomoses, during hypothermic bench surgery, to a Teflon patch by 7–0 polypropylene running suture with a large growth factor

Results

Homogeneous revascularization of the grafted kidney and an immediate urine output were observed in all cases without any bleeding through the vascular anastomotic sites or need for additional stitches; no surgical complications were observed either in the donors or the recipients, but in three patients irreversible acute rejection occurred.

No differences concerning renal function, expressed by the mean value of serum creatinine, or systolic blood pressure were observed between the two groups. The graft survival rate was 89.1 % vs. 88.8 % (control group) at 1 year and 78.5 % vs. 77.4 % (control group) at 5 years. The long-term follow-up color Doppler control, was performed in 40 cases with multiple renal arteries, always showing a normal flow pattern; angiographic studies at different times after transplantation have confirmed these results, excluding arterial stenosis or thrombosis.

Discussion

Living kidney donation has been associated in our experience with no morbidity or mortality in the donor and a very good transplant outcome. The Teflon patch technique that we introduced has proven to be a safe and easy procedure in the presence of multiple renal arteries, allowing prompt homogeneous revascularization and decreasing both the second warm ischemia time and the risk of stenosis or thrombosis.

Moreover, surgical refinement has enabled us to obtain the same satisfactory long-term results as those observed in kidney grafts with normal anatomy, without a greater incidence of surgical complications, thus significantly increasing the pool of potential donors.

Fibrin sealing makes it possible to use a large growth factor, reducing the incidence of anastomotic stenosis, while avoiding adjunctive stitches after revascularization of the graft. Finally, fibrinogen and thrombin, although of human origin, are extremely purified and therefore do not provide immunogenic stimulus, which could increase the risk of graft rejection.

References

1. Berloco P, Alfani D, Cortesini R et al. (1985) Utilization of living donor organs for clinical transplantation. Transplant Proc XVII [Suppl]:3
2. Cortesini R, Berloco P, Alfani D et al. (1988) Long term results in recipients of mismatched related and unrelated living donor kidneys in the cyclosporine age. Transplant Proc XX [Suppl 1]: 41–42
3. Berloco P, Alfani D et al. (1991) Is unrelated living donor a valid organ source in renal transplantation under cyclosporin A therapy? Transplant Proc 23: 912
4. Rossi M, Alfani D, Bruzzone P et al. (1991) Bench surgery for multiple renal arteries in kidney transplantation from living donor. Transplant Proc XXIII (5): 2328–2329
5. Jacob H, Campbell CD, Qiu ZK (1984) Evaluation of fibrin sealing for cardiovascular surgery. Circulation 70 [Suppl 1]: 138–146
6. Alfani D, Berloco P, Cortesini R et al. (1991) Il trapianto di rene: aspetti chirurgici particolari. Il Trapianto Oggi. Atti XXI Congresso della Società Italiana Trapianti d'Organo Milano, pp 105–111

Fibrin Sealing in Surgery of Parenchymal Organs in Adults

M. Schnorrer, J. Pechan, J. Figer, M. Labuda, and I. Makaiová

Abstract

The fibrin glue Tissucol (Immuno, Vienna) was used in organ-preserving surgery of the spleen. Surgical operations on parenchymal organs in adults cause technical problems because of the vulnerability of the tissue. Laceration of puncture channels and section of parenchymal tissue are the most feared complications of the surgical suture. Fibrin gluing as a supplement or even as an alternative to conventional suture techniques enables the general surgeon to repair the organ or perform a tissue-saving operation. During the last 3 years, we have performed partial resection of the spleen due to post-traumatic pseudocyst in three patients. The resected surface was sealed by fibrin sealant. In the postoperative period, spleen regeneration was traced by Tc-99m.

Results in our three patients who underwent operation showed that 30% of the original tissue is sufficient to preserve the complete function of spleen. This report has been prepared for the purpose of presenting results obtained at the authors' hospital using fibrin glue.

Introduction

The first splenectomy was performed in 1559 by Adriano Zaccarelli, and the first partial splenectomy was performed by Viard in 1590 for penetrating injury. In 1881, Billroth described an autopsy finding on the spleen of a patient who died 5 days after injury, on the basis of its characteristics Sherman came to the conclusion that the spleen could have been fully cured [14].

Despite warnings about the importance of the spleen in fighting infections, splenectomies were performed as late as the beginning of the twentieth century. Spleen-preserving treatment was considered hazardous up until then. This opinion began to change when King and Schumaker [8] described overwhelming postsplenectomy infection (OPSI) in children and the first death caused by this infection was published by Coler [2]. Singer [16] critically evaluated 2796 splenectomies from 24 departments. He came to the conclusion that the occurrence of sepsis in children is 100 higher than in the adults. The average interval between surgery and the beginning of sepsis was 4 years (from a minimum of 13 days to a maximum of 14 years). Krivit [9] described OPSI also in congenital aspleny. The frequency of its occurrence was ten times higher than in cases of congenital heart diseases. This was the reason for seeking a way to preserve part or all of the spleen, predominantly after injuries.

Conservative (nonoperative) treatment is influenced by the fact that the spleen is capable of regulating intrasplenic pressure by concentration of arteries, allowing for the creation of thrombi on the injured area. The development of diagnostic methods (ultrasound, computer tomography (CT) scan, nuclear magnetic resonance (NMR) tomography, and gammagraphy) and the possibility of constant monitoring of the general condition of the patient also facilitate the use of nonsurgical methods of treatment [1, 3, 4, 6].

Vital functions must be stabilized and the compensation of the blood volume must not exceed one third. Most of the patients treated in this way are cured, even though secondary cysts can occasionally occur at subcapsular hematomas [12].

Safe hemostasis in the injured areas is becoming the decisive factor, and it is predominantly achieved by using fibrin sealant, ultrasound, and infracoagulation knife [6, 13, 15, 17].

We would like to present our clinical experience with the fibrin sealant Tissucol (Immuno, Vienna) in spleen surgery.

Materials and Methods

During the last 3 years, we have performed partial resection of the spleen due to post-traumatic pseudocyst in three patients.

Case 1: Partial Resection of the Upper Lobe of Spleen

In 1989, splenomegaly with the loss of radioactivity (6.6 × 9.5 cm) was verified by gammagraphy with Tc-99m in a 27-year-old female patient (Fig. 1). In August 1989, surgery was performed under endotracheal anesthesia. After division of the supporting apparatus, the spleen was placed in front of the operation wound (Fig. 2). After ligation of the upper and middle branch of the arteria and vena lienalis and demarcation of tissue, we performed partial resection of the spleen. The resection surface was then treated with the fibrin sealant Tissucol and with suture. The preparation (Fig. 3) had the dimensions 10 × 6 × 6 cm and a calcificated side of 3 mm. On the seventh day after the operation a control gammagraphy was done (Fig. 4), which showed functional remains of the spleen 7.1 × 3.8 cm in size. The postoperative period was without bleeding and other complications.

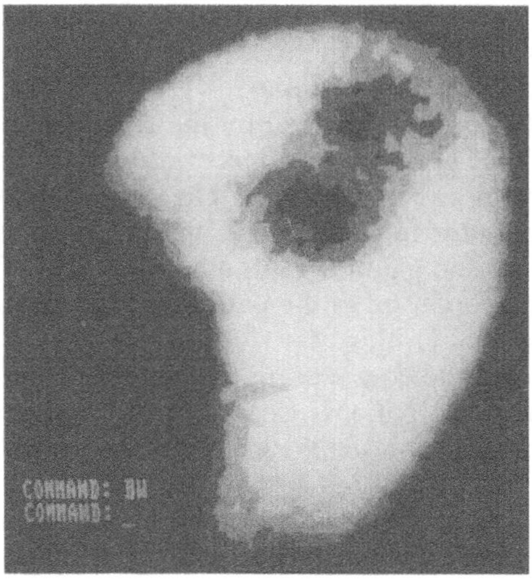

Fig. 1. Preoperative gammagraphy of the spleen with Tc-99m in a female patient, 1962. Spleen has dimensions 11 × 4 × 21.8 cm and shows the loss of radioactivity oval shape, sharply defined, 6.6 × 9.5 cm.

Case 2: Partial Resection of the Lower Lobe of Spleen

In 1991, splenomegaly with the loss of radioactivity (4 × 6 cm) was verified in the lower lobe of spleen by gammagraphy in a 26-year-old female patient (Fig. 5). The pseudocyst on the operative preparation was 7 × 5 cm in size. The resection surface was treated with Tissucol and with suture. No postoperative complications occurred. The control gammagraphy showed the functional remains of spleen 8.3 × 4.8 cm in size (Fig. 6).

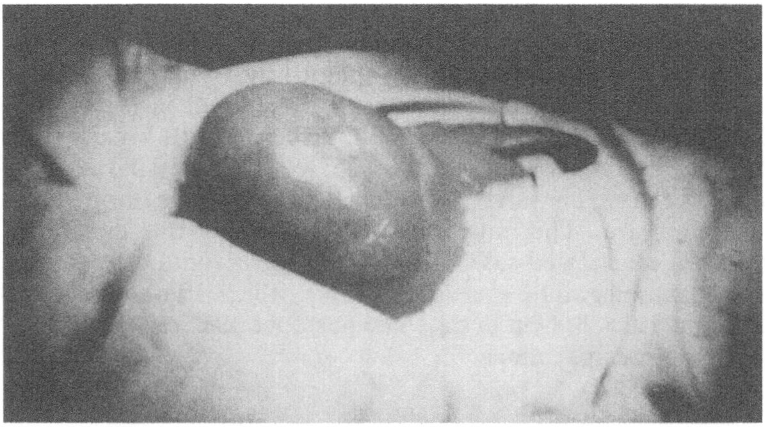

Fig. 2. Perioperative picture after mobilization of the spleen into the operation site in a female patient, 1962. In the upper lobe there is cystic formation of 9 × 6 cm; lower lobe of the spleen is of normal structure

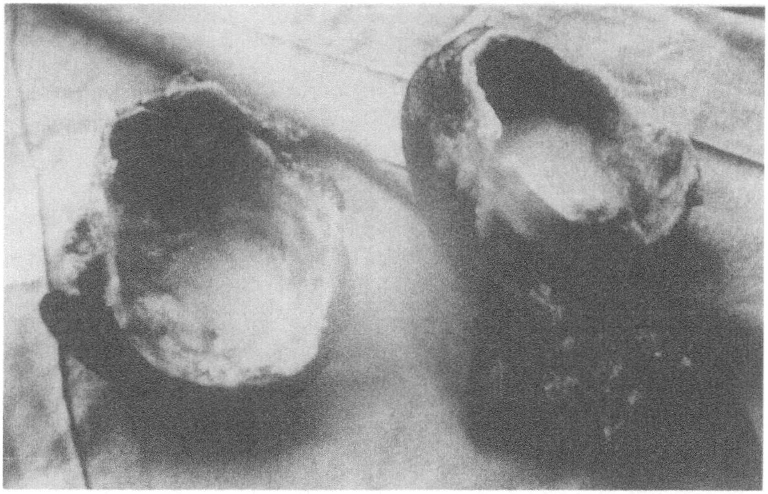

Fig. 3. Preparation of part of spleen in female patient, 1962; cyst after being opened

Case 3: Partial Resection of the Upper Lobe of Spleen

After the injury to the abdominal cavity and recovery from acute pancreatitis, the patient (male, 39-years-old) felt pressure pains under the left rib arc from July 1991 onward. The CT examination showed an extensive pseudocyst of the spleen and the gammagraphy with Tc-99m showed splenomegaly with extensive hypofunctional and afunctional tissue. The patient was operated on 2 December 1991 under endotracheal anesthesia. A pseudocyst of the cauda pancreatis was found. This pseudocyst was filled with hemorrhagic liquid and spanned over the spleen, adhering to its upper pole. The whole pseudocyst was

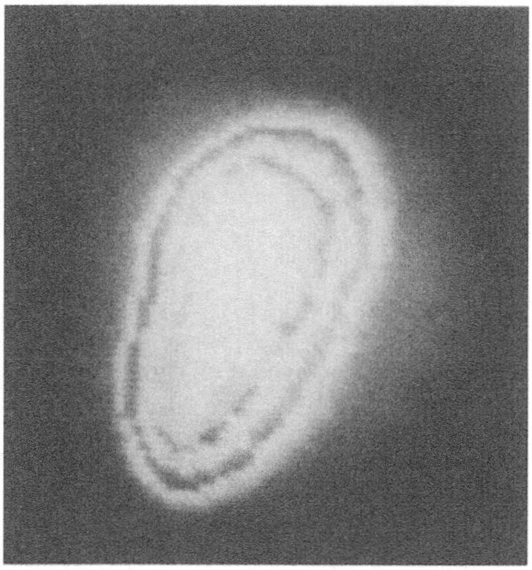

Fig. 4. Postoperative gammagraphy of spleen with Tc-99m in female patient, 1962. Spleen is 7.1 × 3.8 cm in size; note projection of ovoid shape in the anteroposterior and posteroanterior with homogeneous distribution of radioactivity

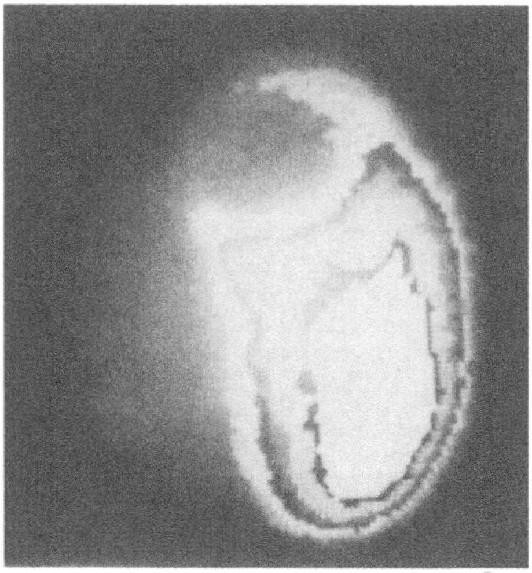

Fig. 5. Preoperative spleen gammagraphy with Tc-99m in female patient, 1965. Loss of radioactivity in 6 × 4 cm in the lower lobe of spleen

removed, requiring partial resection of the upper lobe of the spleen. The resection area was treated with the fibrin sealant Tissucol and with collagen foam. The results of the histological examination confirmed the pseudocyst of the pancreas. The control gammagraphy showed functional remains of the spleen 6.9 × 3.1 cm in size. The postoperative period was without bleeding and other complications.

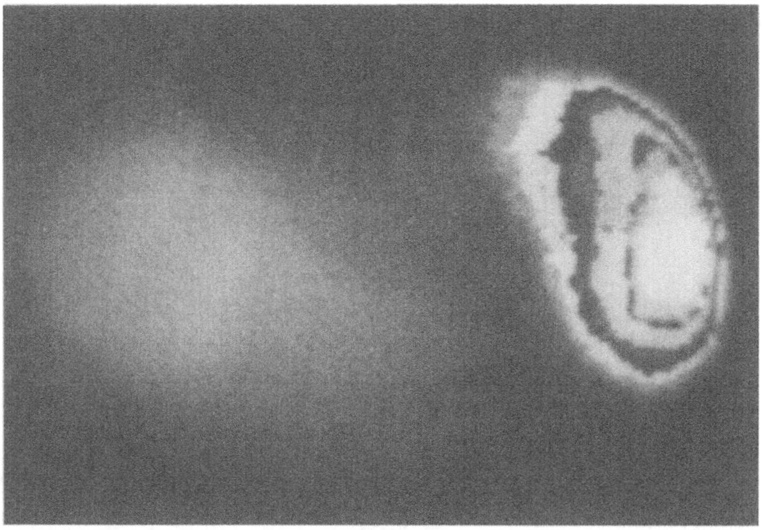

Fig. 6. Patient – woman (1965) Postoperative spleen gammagraphy with Tc-99m in female patient, 1965. Spleen 8.3 × 4.8 cm in size with homogeneous distribution of radioactivity

Results

All the patients were in good condition after the operation, and hematologic, hemocoagulation, and immunologic parameters were within the norm.

The authors refer to the possibilities of preserving part or all of the spleen after injuries or in some diseases, predominantly in pseudocysts or cysts of nonparasital origin. It is necessary to perform a spleen-preserving operation in all cases of spleen injuries. Spleen-preserving surgery using fibrin sealant is of particular significance. The survey was performed using examples of successful treatment of two cases of spleen pseudocyst and one case of intralienal pancreatic pseudocyst. The patients were healed by partial resection of the spleen.

The fibrin sealant Tissucol is well tolerated by tissues; it helps the healing process in general, is highly elastic, absorbs completely, and also has a high hemocoagulative effect. Our experiences prove that it is also of great significance in spleen injuries and resections and assists local hemostasis after splenectomy. Results in our three patients who were operated on showed that 30 % of the original tissue is sufficient to preserve the complete function of spleen.

Discussion

Operative resection of the injured spleen remains the basic and the safest treatment procedure. Splenorrhaphy is most often performed using the mattress stitch and suture of part of the omentum. Fibrin sealants are the most frequently used hemostatic materials. Recently, infrared contact coagulators such as the ultrasound knife have been used for hemostasis. Most of the authors use this procedure in treating spleen injuries. Only a spleen that is completely crushed, separated from hilus, or infected should be indicated for splenectomy.

Ligature of the arteria lienalis and angiographic hemostasis have not been used in clinical practice recently.

Segmental and partial resection of the spleen is determined by its segmental division, as the arteria lienalis is divided into two branches in the hilus. Three branches were found and described by Gupta et al. [5]. The division most often occurs between the cauda pancreatis and hilus of the spleen. In only 10 % of the cases was it found deep in the hilus. Arteria polaris superior and inferior occur in 18 %–80 % of cases. They are of great importance for the surgeon, as they supply the majority of the spleen tissue. In recent years, publications describing spleen resections following injuries have considerably increased. Elective resection of spleen cysts (apart from parasitic ones), benign tumors, intralienal pancreatic cysts, and solitary metastases is indicated (Table 1).

A total of 600 cases of nonparasital cysts have been described in the literature up to now, most of which were of hemorrhagic origin. All of them were treated by splenectomy, and it was not until Sagar and McMahon [12] that two cases of partial splenectomies were described. The cases of spleen resection performed by our surgeons were also followed by gammagraphy. Complete functional capacity of the complex spleen functions has been determined if 25 %–30 % of the original tissue is preserved.

Table 1. Indications for resection of spleen

Therapeutic	Spleen cysts, pseudocysts, benign tumors (splenoma, pulpoma, fibroma), intralienal pancreatic cyst, pseudocysts, solitary metastases
Lesion of spleen	Traumatic (ruptures) Iatrogenic

These findings suggest that in the case of spleen resection, spleen regeneration is favorably influenced by fibrin sealant (Tissucol), postresective necrosis being reduced and the regenerative activity being accelerated in time and volume.

References

1. Buntain WL, Lynn HB (1979) Changing concept for the traumatized spleen. Surgery 86: 747–760
2. Coler RS (1980) Postsplenectomy sepsis. A review of the literature and two new cases. J Trauma 20: 1–13
3. Ein SH, Schnadling N, Simpson JS, Stephans CA (1978) Nonoperative management of traumatized spleen in children: how and why? J Pediatr Surg 13: 117–119
4. Giles RH, Gilday DL, Venogopal S, Schndling B, Asch JM (1978) Splenic trauma nonoperative management and long-term follow-up by scintiscan. J Pediatr Surg 13: 121–126
5. Gupta CD, Aroka AK, Jey R, Sing PA (1976) Vascular segment of the human spleen. J Anat 121: 613–616
6. Hebeler RF, Ward RE, Miller PW, Ben-Menacher Y (1982) Management of splenic injury. J Trauma 22: 492–495
7. Izbicky JR (1990) Existiert ein Sepsissyndrom nach posttraumatischer Splenectomia? Fortschr Med 23: 27–29
8. King H, Schumaker H (1952) Splenic studies. Ann Surg 136: 239–242
9. Krivit W (1977) Overwhelming postsplenectomy infection. Am J Haematol 21: 193–201
10. Kunz E, Buhler R, Gröhling H (1990) Subjektive Folgen des Milzverlustes. Langenbecks Arch Klin Chir 214–219
11. Pearl RH, Wesson DE, Spence LJ et al. (1989) Splenic injury: 5 year update with improved results and changing criteria for conservative management. J Pediatr Surg 24: 428–431
12. Sagar PM, McMahon MJ (1988) Partial splenectomy for splenic cyst. Br J Surg 75: 488–490
13. Seufert RM, Bötther W (1982) Organerhaltende Behandlung von Milzverletzungen, Dtsch Med Wochensch 107: 523–526
14. Sherman NJ (1980) Preoperative perspectives in management of trauma of the spleen. J Trauma 20: 1–13
15. Scheele J (1981) Erste klinische Erfahrungen mit der Fibrinklebung bei traumatischer und intraoperativer Milzverletzung. Chirurg 52: 531–534
16. Singer DB (1973) Postsplenectomy sepsis. Perspect Pediatr 1: 285–311
17. Weltr H (1980) Blutstillung an Leber, Lunge und Milz mittels Infrarotkontaktkoagulator. Zentral Chir 105: 194–201

The Role of Fibrin Sealing in Surgical Treatment of Anal and Perianal Fistulas in Crohn's Disease

P. G. FRIEDL, G. SCHÜRMANN, and Ch. HERFARTH

Abstract

Surgical treatment of perianal or anal fistulas in Crohn's disease depends above all on the activity and pattern of gastrointestinal involvement. Aggressive surgery in high fistulas even with partial division of the sphincter frequently leads to irreversible damage of continence function and is contraindicated in this situation.

With careful local surgery complete long-term success occurs in up to 80 % of simple low fistulas. In 60 %–70 % of high fistulas temporary loop ileostomy, if necessary in combination with local surgical procedures, and fibrin glue application leads to objective improvement of the condition and at least to the absence of symptoms.

Introduction

The anorectal changes in Crohn's disease include lesions of the perianal skin, anal changes and changes in the distal third of the rectum. The incidence of these lesions is largely determinated by the area in which Crohn's disease occurs.

With predominant small bowel involvement, the incidence of anal changes is 8 %–30 %, increasing to 60 %–80 % in cases of large bowel involvement (Table 1). Nearly all patients with involvement of the rectum have perianal manifestations as well.

Results

Analysis of 713 patients with Crohn's disease operated in the Surgical Department of the University of Heidelberg over the past 9 years showed an average of 54 %, with fistulas during that time, this proportion has not changed (Fig. 1). In the series of 452 patients with different types of fistulas, perianal or anal localisation directly follows the interenteric fistulas. With respect to our patient series, the proportion of patients (n = 158) with perianal or anal manifestations is 35 %. A total of 158 patients with perianal fistulas were treated surgi-

Table 1. Perianal Crohn's disease with small- and large-bowel involvement

Authors	Frequency (%)
Small bowel	
Barter (cited in [1])	11.0
Edwards (cited in [1])	12.5
Williams et al. (cited in [1])	14.0
Eckner et al. (cited in [1])	19.5
Kontny (cited in [1])	29.0
Own results (1990)	17.4
Large bowel	
Farmer et al. (cited in [1])	50.0
Williams et al. (cited in [1])	52.0
Wolff et al. [3]	53.4
Fielding (cited in [1])	93.0
Own results (1990)	58.2

cally in 239 procedures (Fig. 2). In nearly half of the patients who underwent resection, diversion of the faeces using loop ileostomy was required. Local procedures such as deroofing, bouginage, or neodymium yttrium aluminium garnet (YAG) – laser coagulation were performed in 74 procedures (Fig. 3). Primary proctectomy was performed in eight patients. In six additional patients, secondary proctectomy was necessary, so the proctectomy rate was 8.8% in relation to the total number of patients in the series. A small group of four

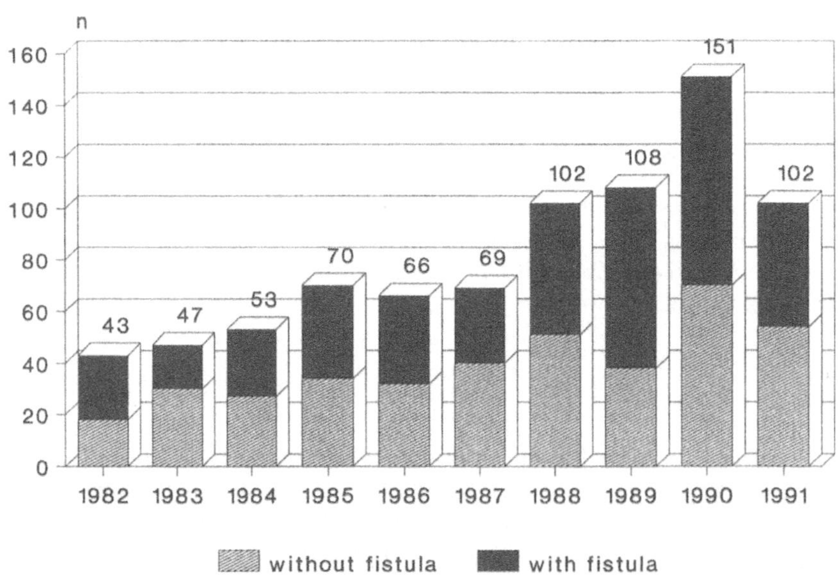

Fig. 1. Number of patients suffering from Crohn's disease (with and without fistulas) operated on at the Surgical University Clinic, Heidelberg, from 1982 to 1991

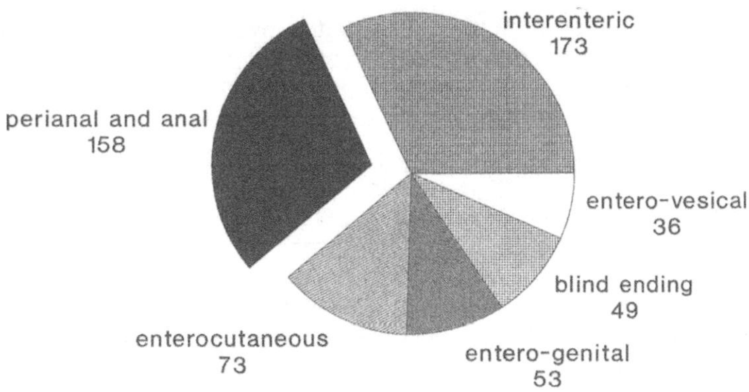

Fig. 2. Types of fistulas in 452 patients with Crohn's disease treated between October 1981 and February 1992

patients with recto-vaginal fistulas and ten patients with high fistulas were treated by mucosal flap plasty and fibrin glue application. In a follow-up period of 1.5 years, nine of 14 patients are free of symptoms. Two patients have asymptomatic recurrent fistulas and one patient had a reoperation of bowel and anal recurrence.

In nine of 69 patients (27.5 %) with temporary loop ileostomy, the stoma was closed after a median interval of 10 months.

The median follow-up period of 34 months shows that in our series, 44 % of the patients develop recurrent Crohn's disease including recurrent fistula (Table 2). According to the literature, the frequency of recurrence depends on the observed time period.

Surgical Treatment

Because of the different clinical therapeutic consequences, Crohn's fistulas are classified as high or low according to their relationship to the sphincter.

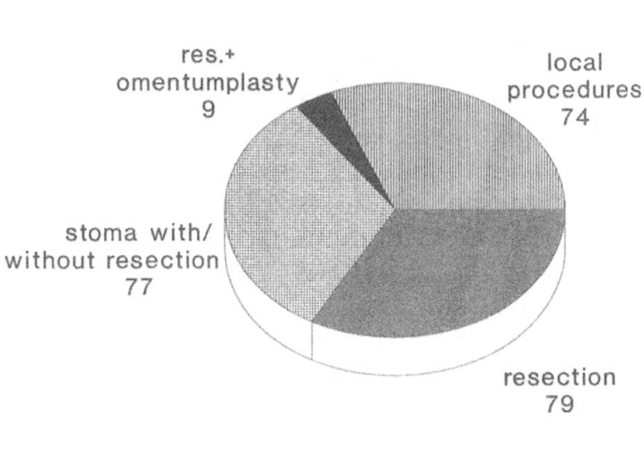

Fig. 3. Surgical treatment of Crohn's perianal fistulas in 158 cases between October 1981 and February 1992. *res.*, resection

Table 2. Long-term results of surgical therapy in anorectal Crohn's disease

Author	Follow-up	Patients (*n*)	Recurrence rate *n*	%
Wolff et al. [3]	26.2 years	84	44	52.4
Levien et al. [2]	82 months	46	27	58.6
Own results (1991)	38 months	34	15	44.0

Low fistulas develop from an infected anal gland, crypt or fissure unusually extended submucosally or occasionally interspincterically from the dentate line to the perianal skin. They are similar to the fistulas seen in the absence of inflammatory bowel disease and may cause symptoms, if any. By contrast, high fistulas develop from transmurally spreading ulcers in the distal rectum, later spreading into the rectal or pelvirectal space. These fistulas are usually symptomatic and progress by destructing the sphincter apparatus or tract towards to the vaginal wall. The indication for surgical treatment should take into account several facts:

1. Surgery is contraindicated in highly inflamed disease (except for treatment of local sepsis).
2. Spontaneous healing of fistulas following resection of bowel segments with active Crohn's disease is reported in the literature. There is, however, a high risk of recurrence.
3. Salvage of the sphincter in high fistulas.

According to the extent of activity and topography of Crohn's lesions, as assessed by endoscopic and radiologic investigations, including magnetic resonance imaging if necessary, the following therapeutic guidelines are to be observed:

1. Non-fistula-dependent careful resection of bowel segments or stricturoplasty in cases with obstructive lesions or foci with inflammation
2. Low fistulas without rectal involvement: deroofing of the fistula tract with excision of granulation tissue; submucosal splitting of the fistula tract with partial internal sphincterotomy
3. Low fistula with rectal involvement: primary deroofing and drainage by seton, the elective situation, closure of the internal opening by flap mobilisation and fibrin glue application
4. High fistula (transsphincteric or extrasphincteric):
   - Deroofing of fistula tracts sparing the sphincter with insertion of a seton
   - Creation of a loop ileostomy for a temporary stoma to divert faeces
   - De-epithelialisation of the fistula tracts with subsequent internal fistula closure by mucosal flap and fibrin glue application
5. Rectovaginal or anovaginal fistulas: excision of the fistula tract from the vaginal approach with separate closure of the rectal and vaginal walls; Loop ileostomy as a temporary stoma for faeces diversion if necessary following individual indications
6. Perianal sepsis with multiple fistula tracts and destruction of the sphincter mechanism: deroofing of the perianal abscess, extirpation of the rectum and proctectomy with sigmoidostomy

References

1. Herfarth C, Bindewald H (1986) Perianale Erkrankung beim M. Crohn. Chirurg 57: 304–308
2. Levien DH, Surell J, Masier WP (1989) Surgical treatment of anorectal fistula in patients with Crohn's disease. Surg Gynecol Obstet 169: 133–136
3. Wolff BG, Culp CE, Beart RW, Ilstrup DM, Ready RL (1985) Anorectal Crohn's disease – a long term perspective. Dis Colon Rectum 28: 709–711

Suggested Reading

4. Alexander-Williams J, Buchmann P (1980) Perianal Crohn's disease. World J Surg 4: 203–207
5. Gross E, Eigler FW (1983) Dic Indikation zur lokal chirurgischen Therapie analer Manifestationen des Morbus Crohn. Langenbecks Arch Chir 75
6. Heyen F, Winslet MC, Andrews H, Alexander-Williams J, Keighley MRB (1989) Vaginal fistulas in Crohn's disease. Dis Colon Rectum 32: 379
7. Post S, Schürmann G, Herfarth C (1990) Das Enterostoma bei Morbus Crohn. Chirurg 62: 306–312
8. Radcliffe AG, Ritchie JK, Hawley PR, Lennard-Jones JE, Northover JM (1988) Anovaginal and rectovaginal fistulas in Crohn's disease. Dis Colon Rectum 31: 94
9. Sohn N, Korelitz BJ, Weinstein MA (1980) Anorectal Crohn's disease: definitive surgery for fistulas and recurrent abscesses. Am J Surg 139: 394–397

Lymphorrhea and Seroma Prevention by Means of Fibrin Glue in Breast and Head and Neck Cancer

L. Moresco, M. Gipponi, G. Canavese, A. Catturich, C. DiSomma, D. Tomei, C. Vecchio, G. Margarino, M. Scala, G. Schenone, P. Meszaros, and F. Badellino

Abstract

Bleeding and lymphorrhea are very frequent side effects in breast cancer (BC) and in head and neck cancer (HNC). They are related to wide muscular resection and/or lymphatic dissection which can delay wound healing in tissue repair. In order to reduce such side effects, between January 1989 and February 1992 two separate groups of patients with BC and HNC underwent intraoperative topical fibrin glue application. In both groups, a reduction in lymphorrhea, wound infection, and, consequently, length of hospitalization was observed as compared to previous experience.

Introduction

Bleeding and lymphorrhea are very frequent side effects in breast cancer (BC) and head and neck cancer (HNC). Such complications are related to wide muscular resection or lymphatic dissection, which can delay wound healing and tissue repair; hence, a proper surgical technique with accurate hemostasis may certainly reduce them, but this is not always sufficient [3, 4].

In this chapter we report our experience with fibrin glue application, which was assessed, as an intraoperative means aimed at reducing bleeding and lymphorrhea and at facilitating cicatrization in patients undergoing BC and HNC surgery.

Methods

Between January 1989 and February 1992, two separate groups of patients with BC and HNC received intraoperative topical fibrin glue application.

A total of 180 patients undergoing BC surgery (100 in treatment group, 80 in control group), were analyzed by daily monitoring of lymphatic drainage. The control group consisted of patients who had been previously investigated in order to show the efficacy of a type of lymph collection tool.

A total of 50 patients in the treatment group and 40 in the control group underwent Patey's modified radical mastectomy; Halsted radical mastectomy

Table 1. Results of the use of fibrin glue in mastectomies

	Patey		Sector		Halsted	
	Treatment group (n = 50)	Control (n = 40)	Treatment group (n = 30)	Control (n = 20)	Treatment group (n = 20)	Control (n = 20)
Tissucol[a] (mean quantity in ml)	8	–	6	–	7	–
Lymphorrhea (ml)	200	325	170	270	170	270
Drainage (days)	4	5	3.5	4	4	5
Wound infection (n)	1	4	1	2	1	2

[a] Immuno, Vienna. Thrombin content, 400–500 IU/ml gas pressure, 4 bar; distance of spray tip from wound surface, 10–20 cm.

was performed in 20 cases in both groups, and sector mastectomy with axillary dissection in 30 and 20 cases, respectively (Table 1). Twelve patients receiving HNC surgery underwent thyroid lobectomy in five cases, near total thyroidectomy in four cases, and radical neck dissection (RND) for laryngeal cancer in

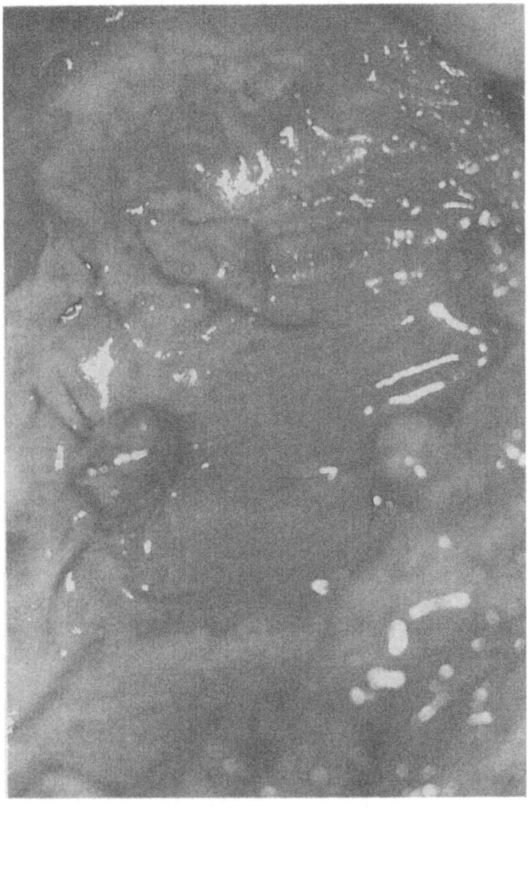

Fig. 1. Tissucol applied by spraying on the chest wall after mastectomy

three cases. In the RND, sternocleidomastoid, muscle, internal jugular vein, and lymphatic tissue, including all five lymph nodes levels, are resected.

In both groups fibrin glue was prepared from four components in two solutions containing 4 and 500 IU thrombin/ml, respectively, and drawn up into separate syringes with subsequent spray application using Duploject (Immuno) on subcutaneous tissue and muscle surface before suction drainage positioning. The gas pressure used was 4 bar. Usually, the distance of the spray head from the wound surface is 10–20 mm (Fig. 1).

After application of fibrin glue, an assistant gently presses the skin flaps toward the underlying wall with his hands (Fig. 2).

Both groups of patients were treated with a mean volume of 7 and 5 ml of biological glue, respectively.

Results

A reduction in lymphorrhea, wound infection and, consequently, the length of hospitalization was observed as compared to previous experience. Overall fluid collection in the treatment and control arms were 190 ml and 325 ml in Patey's mastectomy, 165 ml and 270 ml in Halsted mastectomy, and 160 ml and

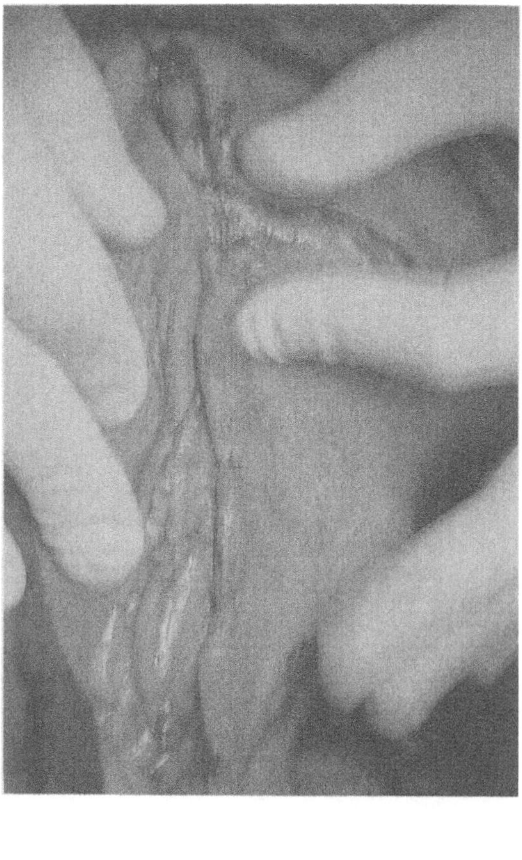

Fig. 2. Radical neck dissection: after application of Tissucol an assistant gently presses the skin flaps toward the deep wall with his hands

270 ml in sector mastectomy, respectively. The mean duration of drainage was 4 versus 5 days in treatment and control patients, respectively (Table 1). Reduction of postoperative bleeding and hematoma was observed as compared to our previous experience. In this group, using 4 IU thrombin, fibrin glue seems to reduce lymphorrhea and bleeding also in patients who underwent preoperative radiotherapy.

Discussion

The use of fibrin sealant (Tissucol, Immuno, Vienna), one of the important technical advances in surgery during the late 1980s, has been advocated to promote hemostasis, adhesion, and wound and tissue repair. Fibrin plays a central role in the physiological process of wound healing. According to examinations by Key [2], fibrin induces the chemotaxis of polymorphonuclear granulocytes and promotes the initial inflammatory phase of the healing process [1, 5]. Wound healing and tissue repair after clot formation begin with the migration of granulocytes and macrophages and are accompanied by capillary sprouting [6, 7].

In our study, these main properties seem to be the biologic background promoting prevention of lymphorrhea and seroma.

According to our experience in HNC and in BC surgery, a good control of lymphorrhea was achieved by adopting the following procedure:

1. Mean dosage of fibrin glue 5–7 ml
2. Thrombin dosage: 4 IU
3. Application by spraying (gas pressure 4 bar)
4. Gentle pression with hands on the skins flaps toward the underlying tissues

The complete knowledge and application of a proper methodology plays a crucial role in achieving the expected results.

Conclusions

Fibrin sealing has now become an accepted tool in many fields of surgery. Our preliminary results suggest that biological fibrin glue can effectively reduce postoperative lymphorrhea, seroma, and hematoma after surgery in BC; it also seems to be beneficial in HNC surgery. A clinical trial is necessary in order to evaluate the real impact of fibrin glue on the prevention of postoperative lymphorrhea and bleeding.

References

1. Giardino R, Fini M (1990) I collanti in chirurgia. Proc SIATEC VI: 495–503
2. Key AB, Pepper DS, Ewart MR (1973) Generation of chemotactic activity for leukocytes by the action of thrombin on human fibrinogen. Nature 243: 56–57
3. Moresco L (1989) Impiego del Tissucol nella chirurgia del cancro mammario. Proc SIATEC V: 567–569
4. Moresco L, Scala M, Canavese G, Bertoglio S, Cafiero f (1988) Il collante biologico in chirurgia oncologica. Proc SICO XII: 599–603
5. Redl H, Schlag G (1986) Fibrin sealant and its modes of application. Fibr Seal Op Med 6: 13–26
6. Redl H, Schlag G, Dinges HP (1985) The use and biocompatibility of a human fibrin sealant for hemostasis and tissue sealing. Biocomp Tissue Tissue Analog 1: 136–157
7. Schlag G, Redl H, Turnher M, Dinges HP (1986) The importance of fibrin in wound repair. Fib Seal Op Med 6: 3–12

Prevention and Treatment of Lymphatic Fistulae with Fibrin Sealing Following Lymph Node Dissections

H. W. Waclawiczek and O. Boeckl

Abstract

Lymph node dissections in the axillary or inguinal regions and after vascular procedures are frequently complicated by lymphoceles or lymphatic fistulae even under optimal operative conditions. Such lymph fistulae occur mainly after radical lymphadenectomies in the surgical treatment of malignant tumors. An incidence of up to 35 % must be considered. This complication, although uncomfortable, does not carry any immediate danger to the patient. However, in the long run, there is an increased risk of infection. Until recently, only sharp dissections and ligations of the larger and visible lymph vessels along with the drainage of the wound area were available to prevent lymph seromas. With the use of fibrin sealing (FS), it is now possible to permanently occlude even the smaller, invisible lymph vessels. Even an already existing lymphocele can be treated successfully.

Between 1984 and June 1992, 138 patients underwent radical lymph node dissections in the axillary ($n = 76$) and/or inguinal ($n = 62$) region, which were carried out by isolating and ligating the larger lymph vessels. Before skin closure and drainage, the whole wound area was additionally sealed with a thin layer of fibrin glue. By using the Duploject application set with the attached spray head (Tissomat), wide distribution and better use of the quantity of FS could be achieved. On average, 1 ml FS was sufficient.

In 20 cases of an existing lymphatic fistula, the wound cavity was punctured percutaneously and the lymphatic juice was aspirated completely. The FS was applied via the same puncture needle (1–2 ml). Of importance was the subsequent compression of the wound area for at least 10 min. In larger lymphoceles, the above procedure was repeated up to three times.

In a prospective randomized study, only one case of postoperative seroma (3.8 %) occurred in the patients who underwent fibrin sealing ($n = 26$). In the control group, the complication rate was considerably higher (15.4 %). The duration and quantity of postoperative lymph secretion through the drain was significantly reduced in the group using FS. Until June 1992, prophylactic fibrin sealing was performed in 112 additional patients. We observed only three more cases of postoperative lymphatic fistulae (2.6 %).

In 18 out of 20 patients with evident postoperative lymphatic fistulae, the treatment with FS was successful. In eight cases one, in seven cases two, and in five cases three applications of FS were necessary. In two cases a redon drainage had to be applied until the lymph flow had stopped. These two patients were among those treated during the initial use of this method, when repeated application of FS had not yet been considered. Prophylactic as well as therapeutic use of FS is technically simple and requires only a short time. Therefore, it can be recommended for routine use. Of course, the cost factor is considerable, but is justified by shortened treatment time and hospital stay for patients.

Introduction

Lymph node dissections in the inguinal or axillary regions and after vascular procedures are frequently complicated by lymphoceles or lymphatic fistulae even under optimal operative conditions. Such lymphatic fistulae appear mainly after radical lymphadenectomies in the surgical treatment of carcinomas (breast carcinoma, melanoma, soft tissue sarcoma). According to a report by Tonak et al. [3], an incidence of 15–43 % must be considered: the inguinal region is afflicted more frequently. This complication, although uncomfortable, does not carry any immediate danger to the patient. However, in the long run there is an increased risk of infection [1,3, 4].

The accumulation of lymph produces an ideal culture medium for pathogenic bacteria. In addition, drains must be maintained to treat a lymphatic fistula, thus again promoting infections. Until recently, only sharp dissection and ligations of the larger and visible lymph vessels along with drainage of the wound area were available to prevent lymph seromas. With the use of fibrin sealing, it is now possible to permanently occlude even the smaller, invisible lymph vessels. Even an already existing lymphocele can be treated successfully. The efficiency of this new prophylactic and therapeutic method was examined in a prospective randomized study [5].

Methods and Patients

Prophylaxis

Between 1982 and 1992, 194 patients (108 axillary lymph node dissections, 86 inguinal lymph node dissections) underwent the following treatment: radical lymph node dissection was always performed, observing generally accepted oncosurgical principles (e.g., axilla, levels I and II). Dissection was carried out mainly using a scalpel and scissors, with special emphasis on tissue preservation. Larger lymph vessels were isolated and ligated with absorbable sutures (4–0 Vicryl; polyglactin 910). Electrocoagulation was used as rarely as possible. Before skin closure, the whole wound area was additionally sealed with a thin layer of fibrin glue (Fig. 1).

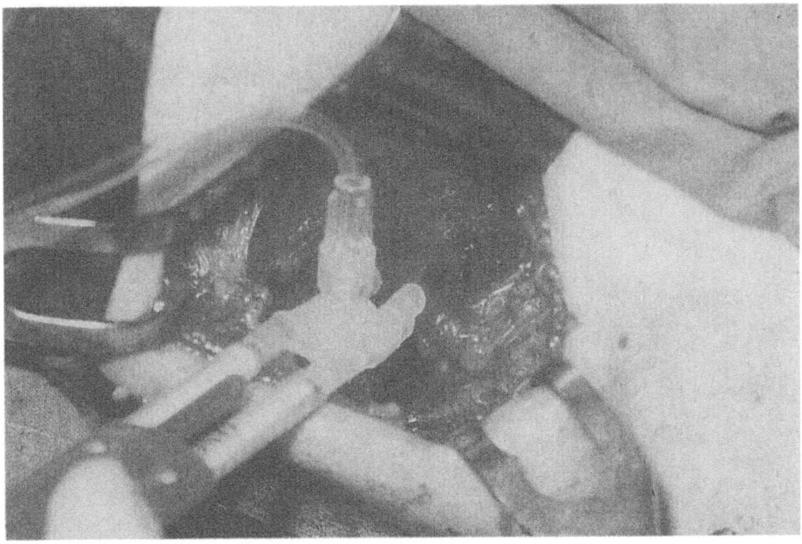

Fig. 1. Sealing of the wound area (axilla) with a thin fibrin film using a spray head

By using the Duploject application set (Immuno, Vienna) with the attached spray head, combined with an air pump and sterile filter (Tissomat, Immuno, Vienna), wide distribution and better use of the quantity of fibrin sealant could be achieved [2]. On average, 1 ml fibrin sealant was sufficient (Tissucol. Immuno, Vienna).

Due to the high fibrinolytic activity of lymph, a high concentration of aprotinin (5000 IU/ml) was used. The high thrombin content (500 IU/ml) supported the rapid solidification of the sealant. All wounds were drained using a vacuum drainage system.

In a prospective randomized study, 26 patients were treated with fibrin sealant between September 1983 and June 1985. Indications for lymph node dissection in the axilla were breast carcinomas (n = 6) or melanomas of the upper extremities (n = 3), and in the inguinal region, melanomas (n = 15) or soft tissue sarcomas (n = 2) of the lower extremities. The control group (n = 26) was comparable concerning the indications for lymph node dissection (five breast carcinomas, 20 melanomas, one soft tissue sarcoma), the distribution in the axillary (n = 9) and the inguinal (n = 17) region, and the above-mentioned, technical criteria. However, no fibrin sealant was added in this control group. The average age in the group with fibrin sealant was 48.7 years, and in the control group 50.6 years. All operations were performed by the same two surgeons.

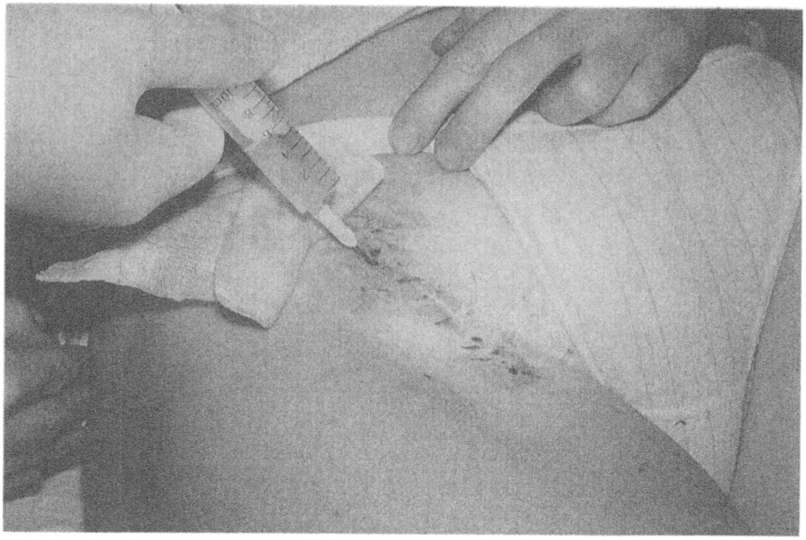

Fig. 2. Punction of the lymphocele and aspiration of lymphatic juice

Therapy

In the 20 cases of an existing lymphocele or lymphatic fistula, the wound cavity was punctured percutaneously and the lymphatic juice was aspirated completely (Fig. 2). The fibrin sealant was applied via the same puncture needle (1 ml average; Fig. 3). Of importance is the subsequent compression of the wound

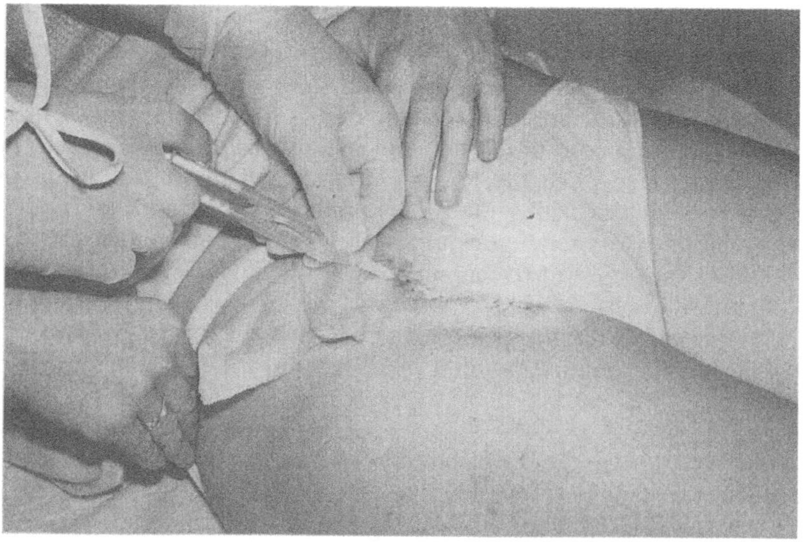

Fig. 3. Application of fibrin sealant through the puncture needle

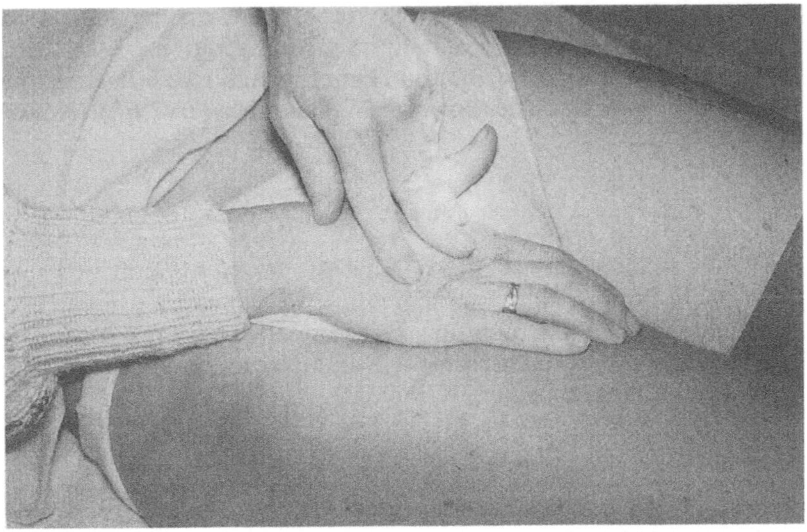

Fig. 4. Digital compression of the wound area for about 10 min

area for at least 10 min (Fig. 4). In the larger lymphoceles, the above procedure was repeated several times, each time resulting in a smaller cavity until the lymphocele was dissolved.

Results

Prophylaxis

In the course of the prospective randomized study, only one case of a postoperative seroma (3.8 %) occurred in the patients who underwent fibrin sealing. In the control group, the complication rate was considerably higher (15.4 %). The duration and quantity of postoperative lymph secretion through the drains were significantly reduced in the group with fibrin sealant as compared to the control group (Table 1).

Table 1. Additional fibrin sealing of wound regions following lymph node dissections

Group	Postoperative lymph drainage		Presence of lymph fistulae	
	Duration (days)	Quantity (ml)	(*n*)	(%)
Fibrin sealing (n = 26)	1.8	23 ± 10	1	3.8
Control (n = 26)	4.7	105 ± 35	4	15.4

Until December 1992, prophylactic fibrin sealing was performed in 168 additional patients. We observed only four additional cases of postoperative lymphatic fistulae. Thus, the total lymph fistula rate following lymph node dissection and prophylactic fibrin sealing amounted to 2.6% (five out of 194).

Therapy

In 18 out of 20 patients with evident postoperative lymphatic fistulae, the treatment with fibrin sealant was successful. In two cases, a redon drainage had to be applied until the lymph flow had stopped. These two cases occurred during the initial stage of this treatment, when repeated application of fibrin sealant had not yet been considered (Table 2).

Table 2. Number of fibrin sealant applications and results in lymph fistulae following lymph node dissections with fibrin sealing

Fibrin sealant applications	Successful (*n*)	Ineffective (*n*)	Total (*n*)
1	4	2	6
2	9	0	9
3	5	0	5
Total	18	2	20

Discussion

Lymphatic fistulae or lymphoceles do not represent serious complications in carcinoma surgery, but are annoying for both the patient and the concerned physician. In vascular surgery they are especially dangerous, because the risk of infection of artificial grafts must be taken into consideration.

Delayed wound healing and prolonged treatment result in additional stress for the patient.

To avoid postoperative lymphatic fistulae, a very sharp, tissue-sparing dissection with ligation of the larger lymph vessels is still essential. If possible, blunt mobilization with fingers or coagulation in the axilla should be avoided. By means of fibrin sealing even the smallest lymph vessels can now be occluded [5]. This fact was confirmed by our prospective randomized study, in which duration as well as quantity of lymphatic secretion was significantly reduced due to the use of fibrin sealing [5]. The complication rate was reduced to 2.6% (five out of 194). In an already existing lymphatic fistula, successful treatment can be performed using fibrin sealing. It should also be taken into account that this method can be repeated at will and that especially the large lymphoceles can close permanently after repeated use of fibrin sealing. The choice of high concentrations of aprotinin and thrombin is of special importance because of the high fibrinolytic activity of the lymph. Again, it should be pointed out that compression of the wound area for at least 10 min or, better still, the employment of pressure bandages is mandatory.

If all the described measures are taken, the fibrin sealing method can be expected to succeed. In addition, conjugate therapeutic measures (mainly radiotherapy, performed obligatorily after reduced radical mammary gland surgery) can be started earlier.

Prophylactic as well as therapeutic use of fibrin sealing is technically simple and requires only a short time. Thus, it can be recommended for routine use. Of course, the cost factor is considerable, but is justified by a shortened treatment and hospital stay for the patient.

References

1. Kubik S (1981) Chirurgische Anatomie des Lymphsystems. In: Hennigsen B (ed) Lymphologische Probleme in der Chirurgie. EBM, Munich
2. Seelich T, Redl H (1984) Applikationstechniken. In: Scheele J (ed) Fibrinklebung. Springer. Berlin Heidelberg New York, pp 11–16
3. Tonak J, Gall FP, Hoferichter S (1981) Chirurgische Komplikationen der regionalen Lymphknotendissektion. Krebsmedizin 2: 112
4. Tonak J, Gall FP, Hermanek P (1983) Die chirurgische Therapie von Lymphknotenmetastasen: Hals, Axilla, Leiste, Chirurg 54: 561
5. Waclawiczek HW, Pimpl W (1986) Lymphfisteln nach Lymphknotendissektionen – Verhütung und Behandlung mit Hilfe der Fibrinklebung. Chirurg 57: 330

Tissue Adhesives in Experimental Intestinal Anastomoses

M. FINI, R. GIARDINO, G. GIAVARESI, M. ROCCA, and N. N. ALDINI

Abstract

The aim of this study was to investigate the effects of a synthetic and a biological glue in intestinal anastomoses healing processes. An experimental model was also adopted for evaluating the possible side effects linked to fibrin glue use which are reported in different studies on colonic anastomoses. Twenty male New Zealand white rabbits (b. w. 3 ± 0.350 kg) under general anaesthesia were used. Animals were divided into three groups of six rabbits each and in two animals sham operation was performed. In 18 animals 5 cm of the left colon was resected by midline laparotomy. The anastomoses were performed using three different techniques: group I, single-layer end-to-end anastomosis with interrupted 6–0 polyglycolic acid stitches, group II: four 6–0 polyglycolic acid stitches at the cardinal points plus butyl-2-cyanoacrylate; and in group III, four 6–0 polyglycolic acid stitches at the cardinal points plus fibrin glue. Animals were killed under general anaesthesia at days 7, 14 and 21 for macroscopic and histologic analysis.

No intra- or post-operative complications were observed. In group I, three cases of perianastomotic granuloma were observed, and in two animals modest adhesion formation was found. In group II, adhesion formation was evident and, moreover, one animal at day 7 had an anastomotic leakage. In the same group, two cases of a macroscopically evident stenosis of the anastomosis were observed at day 14. In group III, no macroscopical complications were noticed. With histologic study the anastomoses that had healed best were the ones in groups I and III, while in group II superficial necrosis of the perivisceral adipose tissue occurred.

The results show the possibility of performing intestinal anastomoses with glues at least in experimental conditions. Moreover, anastomoses performed with biological glue seem to be more reliable and have less side effects.

Introduction

Intestinal anastomoses can be performed with traditional or mechanical sutures. These techniques require the use of a great amount of materials and, even if they possess a certain biocompatibility, some negative tissue reactions can occur. Moreover, these materials must be considered as foreign bodies, which could interfere with normal healing processes.

Previous comparative in vitro and in vivo studies have been performed in our department on suture materials, and the results of these tests have shown that all of them can cause a certain inflammatory response [1–4, 8]. The use of different glues could contribute to the reduction or even the substitution of suture materials in intestinal anastomosis.

These aims led us to perform a study to compare different materials in intestinal anastomoses: traditional suture materials and two commercially available sealants, synthetic butyl-2-cyanoacrylate and biological fibrin glue.

Materials and Methods

Butyl-2-cyanoacrylate is a cyanoacrylate with better properties than the others in the same family. It possesses a high molecular weight and offers various advantages: hydrocyanic radical esterification occurs with substances from the butyl group and causes hydrocarbonate chain elongation and, consequently, a great reduction in toxicity. It undergoes quick polymerization, has a proportionately brief absorption time, less viscosity, good elasticity and plasticity, with an important adhesive capability.

Human fibrin glue contains human fibrinogen and factor XIII (75 mg/ml) and is added to a solution containing thrombin and calcium dichloride. The resulting mixture mimics the final steps of the coagulation process.

Twenty male New Zealand white rabbits (b. w. 3 ± 0.350 kg) were anaesthetized by subcutaneous ketamine (25 mg/kg)) and xylazine (2 mg/kg) injection and maintained under alothane and O_2 by automatic ventilation. Two rabbits were then subjected to laparotomy only (sham operations) and in 18 rabbits, 5 cm of left colon was resected. The intestinal continuity with an end-to-end anastomosis was restored using three different techniques:

Group I (six animals), extramucosal single layer with 14–16 interrupted 6–0 polyglycolic acid stitches; group II (six animals), four interrupted 6–0 polyglycolic acid stitches at the cardinal points plus butyl-2-cyanoacrylate; group III (six animals), four interrupted 6–0 polyglycolic acid stitches at the cardinal points plus human fibrin glue.

Two animals per group were killed under general anaesthesia at days 7, 14 and 21 for determining macroscopic and histologic findings.

This study was carried out in conformity with the International Guiding Principles for Biomedical Research Involving Animals and Italian Rules.

Results

No intraoperative deaths or postoperative complications were observed.

In group I, three cases of perianastomotic granuloma were observed (Fig. 1) and two animals presented modest adherences between intestinal loops

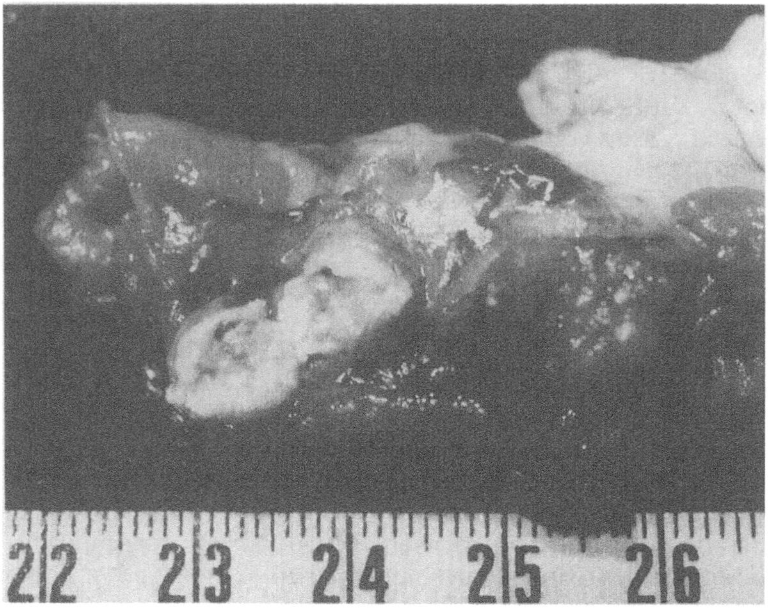

Fig. 1. Macroscopic findings: great perianastomotic granuloma in suture material group at day 21

around the anastomoses. In group II, four animals showed great and tenacious adherences (Fig. 2). One of these animals had a covered and partial leakage in the posterior wall of the intestinal anastomosis at day 7. In two rabbits which were killed at day 14, a serious anastomotic stenosis was found. In group III, no macroscopical complications were observed.

Histological analysis confirmed the macroscopic data: the anastomoses that had healed best were found in the suture material and particularly in fibrin glue groups (Fig. 3). Anastomoses performed with butyl-2-cyanoacrylate showed in some cases superficial necrosis in the perivisceral adipose tissue and vascular intramural thrombosis. A foreign body granulomatosis reaction surrounded suture materials.

Discussion

Colorectal surgery still causes quite a large amount of complications, probably due to the particular visceral content. Indeed, despite the obtained improvements concerning suture material biocompatibility, the advanced preparation techniques in colon surgery, the availability of mechanical staplers and the effectiveness antibiotic prophylaxis [7], anastomotic complications are still observed.

The haemostatic, waterproofing and sealing properties of synthetic and biological glues could remarkably decrease intestinal anastomotic complications.

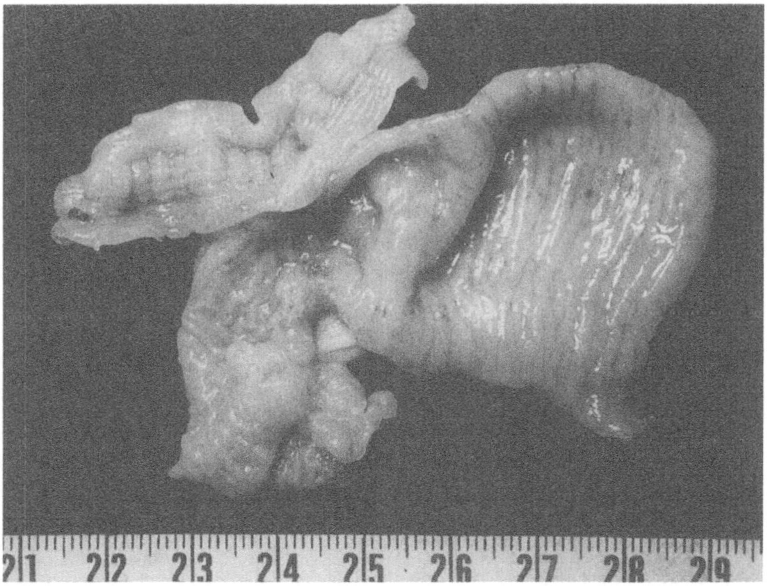

Fig. 2. Macroscopic findings: conspicuous stenosis of the anastomosis with a tenacious adhesion formation with an ileal loop in butyl-2-cyanoacrylate group at day 14

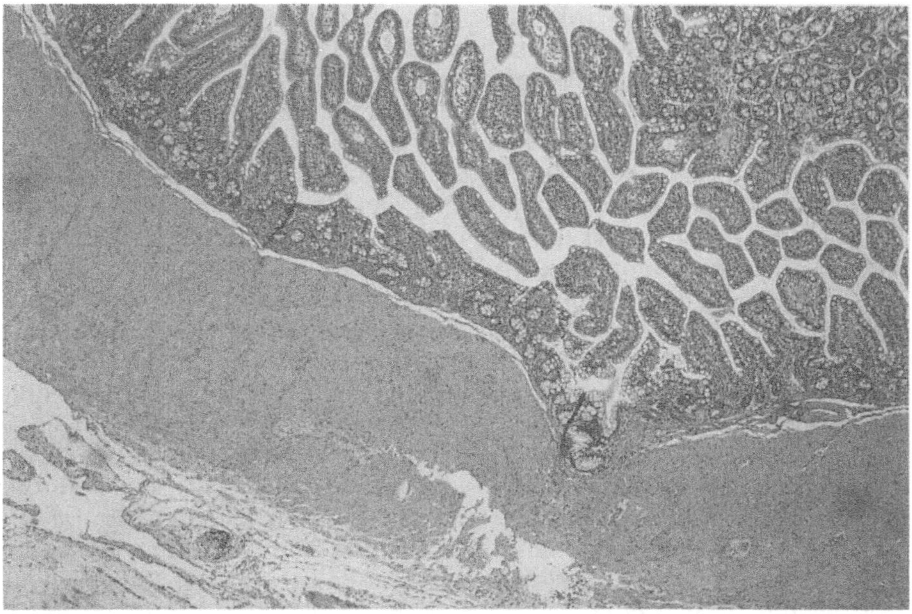

Fig. 3. The anatomical layers at anastomosis level show a regular healing process in the absence of inflammatory reaction in the fibrin glue group at day 21

We performed a comparative experimental study between synthetic (butyl-2-cyanoacrylate) and biologic (fibrin glue) sealants.

The former have been known and experimented with for a long time. Since 1960, a preliminary group of synthetic substances (ioplex, methacrylate, etc.) has been evaluated for surgical applications, and as a result of the difficult handling and the serious toxicity of this first group of substances, they have been substituted by newer sealants such as methyl-2-cyanoacrylate, butyl-2-cyanoacrylate and isobutyl-cyanoacrylate [13]. Butyl-2-cyanoacrylate is the one that has been most widely tested and used, thanks to its low toxicity, good holding and adhesion.

Fibrin glue also has many surgical applications and experimentally it is employed to perform colorectal anastomoses [6]. The comparison between the two different glues and the evaluation of these preliminary results show the good reliability of this experimental model and also the fact that intestinal anastomoses performed using fibrin glue are safer than the ones made with synthetic sealant. In fact, in experimental conditions, complications due to material histotoxicity were not observed in the fibrin glue group, while butyl-2-cyanoacrylate caused tissue necrosis and, consequently, difficult intestinal anastomosis healing.

We emphasize that the use of fibrin glue in intestinal anastomoses did not show macroscopic or histologic side effects on days 7, 14 and 21 in our experimental study. These results agree with our clinical experience [5]. Other experimental studies by different authors provided negative results on fibrin glue in abdominal surgery in rats with adhesions, leakages or abscess formation. These results are explained by the natural contamination of anastomosis and fibrin, which acts as a culture medium for pathogens. Infection and inflammatory reaction around the anastomosis could influence the collagenase activity, with a consequent degradation of collagen followed by a decrease in anastomotic strength [9, 12]. Our study gave better results in the fibrin glue group than in the synthetic glue and suture material group. In fact, some differences exist between the experimental models: in our study, the number of stitches was smaller in fibrin glue anastomoses than in others, and it is important to observe that suture biomaterials could also cause tissue reactions due to either a foreign body reaction or bacterial adhesion [8]. Moreover, some authors recognize the importance of the site and the tension of sutures in early breaking strength in intestinal anastomoses, and they suggest the importance of proteinases of neutrophil origin in collagen degradation. The proteinase amount did not change, while at the same time there were pronounced differences in anastomotic breaking strength, so one has to consider the systemic mechanism of protection against proteinase action. A great number of stitches, different tension or distance from the anastomosis cut edges could reduce blood flow at the bowel edge, with a decrease in serum proteinase inhibitors [10, 11]. Thus, it could be possible that fibrin is not directly responsible for collagen disruption in models in which too many suture stitches are used and in which there is too much mechanical stress on the anastomosis during the first 4 days of healing.

Finally, some unresolved problems arise for other surgical techniques as well as for intestinal anastomoses with fibrin glue, and we think that understanding the role and effectiveness of fibrin glue in abdominal surgery requires other experimental studies with a standardization of experimental models.

Acknowledgement. This research was supported by grants from the Istituti Ortopedici Rizzoli, Ricerca Corrente, area 2.

References

1. Arciola CR, Buscaroli S, Rocca M, Farinetti A, Fini M, Manfrini M, Giardino R (1990) Studio in vitro sull'adesività dello stafilococco epidermidis sui fili da sutura. Chir XI (3): 141–143
2. Buscaroli S, Arciola CR, Mancini I, Farinetti A, Fini M, Rocca M, Giardino R (1990) Influenza dei materiali da sutura sulla vitalità cellulare: studio comparativo sperimentale. G Chir XI (3): 147–148
3. Buscaroli S, Ciapetti G, Fini M, Rocca M, Giardino R (1990) T Lymphocytes activation and soluble receptor interleukin 2 release by biomedical polymers. Int J Artif Organs 13(9): 594
4. Buscaroli S, Stea S, Arciola CR, Rocca M, Nicoli Aldini N, Fini M, Mancini M, Giardino R (1990) Il burst ossidativo per la determinazione della risposta immunitaria ai materiali di sintesi. G Chir XI (3): 144–146
5. Giardino R, Brulatti M, Franchini A (1986) Colonic anastomoses protected with fibrin sealant. In: Schlag G, Redl H. General surgery and abdominal surgery. Springer, Berlin Heidelberg New York, pp 155–158 (Fibrin sealant in operative medicine, vol 6)
6. Giardino R, Ussia G, Grilli Cicilioni C, Salerno A, Feldmann D, Farruggia F, Galletti G (1986) Colo-rectal anastomoses with fibrin sealant and transmural approaching device in pig. Eur Surg Res 18 [Suppl 1/86]
7. Giardino R (1987) La profilassi antibiotica in chirurgia. Bazzi, Milano
8. Giardino R, Rocca M, Fini M, Buscaroli S, Arciola CR, Nicoli Aldini N, Morrone G (1992) Adesività batterica e reattività tessutale dei materiali per la sintesi: studio sperimentale in vitro ed in vivo. G. Chir XIII (4): 248–249
9. Houston G, Rotstein OD (1988) Fibrin sealant in high-risk colonic anastomoses. Arch Surg 123: 230–234
10. Jonsson T, Hogstrom H (1991) Neutrophil-dependent decrease in early wound margin strength. Arch Surg 126: 1423–1426
11. Jonsson T, Hogstrom H (1992) Effect of suture technique on early healing of intestinal anastomoses in rats. Eur J Surg 158: 267–270
12. Van der Ham AC, Kort WJ, Weijma IM, van der Ingh HFGM, Jeekel H (1992) Effect of antibiotics in fibrin sealant on healing anastomoses in the rats. Br J Surg 79: 525–528
13. Woodward SC et al.(1965) Histotoxicity of cyanoacrylate tissue adhesive in the rat. Ann Surg 162: 113–122

Submucosal Fibrin Adhesion in Upper Gastrointestinal Bleeding

J. LABENZ, U. PEITZ, M. WIECZOREK, and G. BÖRSCH

Abstract

During the past 15 years, several methods of endoscopic hemostasis have been evaluated in clinical studies, for injection therapy with adrenalin/polidocanol. However, these substances may produce tissue damage. In some pilot studies, excellent results concerning initial and definitive control of peptic ulcer hemorrhage were obtained with submucosal injection of a fibrin tissue adhesive.

In the past 2½ years, 83 patients with upper gastrointestinal (GI) bleeding – peptic ulcer hemorrhage, $n = 68$ (Forrest I a, $n = 16$; I b, $n = 20$; II a, $n = 29$; II b, $n = 3$); Mallory-Weiss tear, $n = 3$; varices, $n = 3$; esophageal ulcer/esophagitis, $n = 4$; angiodysplasia, $n = 2$; gastric carcinoma, $n = 1$; and sphincterotomy bleeding, $n = 2$ – diagnosed endoscopically were treated with a two-component fibrin adhesive (Tissucol Duo S, Immuno, Heidelberg, Germany) via a double lumen catheter. Initial control of bleeding was achieved in 96.4% (80/83) of patients. Early rebleeding occurred in 11 out of 80 patients (13.8%), which could be effectively managed by repeated injection of the fibrin adhesive in six patients. Nine patients (10.8%) required emergency ($n = 5$) or elective surgery ($n = 4$). The overall mortality rate was 6.0%. Complications due to submucosal injection of the fibrin adhesive were not observed.

In conclusion, endoscopic submucosal injection of a fibrin adhesive was highly effective (96.4% of patients) in initial control of upper GI hemorrhage predominantly due to peptic ulcer bleeding. By including repeated injections, definitive hemostasis was achieved in 90.4%. Prospective, randomized, and controlled studies are necessary to confirm these encouraging results.

Introduction

During the past 15 years, several methods for endoscopic treatment of gastrointestinal bleeding (GI), have been evaluated in clinical studies and proved to be highly successful with regard to initial control of bleeding and reduction of bleeding relapses, frequency of surgical interventions, and mortality [3]. The hemostatic mechanisms included local edema and reduction of blood flow induced by vasoconstrictives and thermic (electro- and laser-coagulation, heater probe) or chemical lesions (e.g., polidocanol) of the tissue [8].

Most endoscopists now prefer sclerotherapy, because this method is easy to learn, practicable everywhere, cheap, and of equal efficiency compared with the other methods mentioned above. However, the injected sclerosants produce tissue damage, entailing the risk of rebleeding and severe complications [2, 7].

Fibrin sealant seems to be a suitable substance for transendoscopic injection therapy, because it combines efficient initial hemostasis and the first step of wound healing (substrate phase) without additional damage of tissue. Fibrin sealant was superior to polidocanol in experimental studies with Wistar rats [8], and excellent results concerning initial and definitive hemostasis were obtained in some pilot studies in humans with upper GI bleeding predominantly due to peptic ulcer hemorrhage [4, 6, 8].

Patients and Methods

In the past 3 years, 100 patients with upper GI bleeding of various etiology were endoscopically treated with submucosal or intravariceal injection of 1–2 ml of a two-component fibrin tissue adhesive (Tissucol Duo S, Immuno, Heidelberg, Germany) via a double lumen catheter. In some patients with active peptic ulcer bleeding or visible vessel, 4–10 ml adrenaline (1:10000) was additionally injected in the surroundings of the bleeding lesion. All patients also received omeprazole or ranitidine intravenously. Re-endoscopies were performed within the next 24 h or when recurrent bleeding was suspected clinically. Lesions with active rebleeding or visible vessel were again treated as described above.

Results

The indications for submucosal fibrin adhesion comprised bleeding from peptic ulcers ($n = 80$), Mallory-Weiss tears ($n = 6$), esophageal ulcers/esophagitis ($n = 5$), angiodysplasias ($n = 3$), esophageal, fundic, and duodenal varices ($n = 3$), sphincterotomy wound ($n = 2$), and gastric carcinoma ($n = 1$). An overview of treatment results is given in Table 1.

Initial hemostasis was achieved in all but one patient with active bleeding from duodenal or gastric ulcers ($n = 41$). In one patient with arterial bleeding from an ulcer at the posterior wall of the duodenal bulb, injection therapy failed to induce hemostasis. A bleeding relapse was observed in 12 patients with peptic ulcers, which was effectively managed by repeated injections of fibrin sealant in seven patients. Emergency ($n = 5$) or early elective surgery ($n = 3$) was done in eight patients (Table 2).

Hemostasis without evidence of a bleeding relapse was achieved in all patients with hemorrhage due to Mallory-Weiss tear, esophageal ulcer or esophagitis, and angiodysplasia. Intravascular injection of fibrin adhesive primarily

Table 1. Overview of clinical results of endoscopic hemostasis by injection of fibrin sealant in 100 patients

	Number of patients	Percentage
Initial success of fibrin sealant	97/100	97
Recurrent bleeding	14/ 97	14.4
Definitive hemostasis by fibrin sealant	87/100	87
Sclerotherapy with polidocanol or Histoacryl	3/100	3
Emergency surgery	6/100	6
Early elective surgery	3/100	3
Elective surgery	1/100	1
Mortality (30 days)	6/100	6

failed in two patients with esophageal and fundic variceal hemorrhage, respectively. A bleeding relapse from a duodenal varix several days after successful control with fibrin sealant was definitely cured by endoscopic embolization with Histoacryl (Braun-Melsungen). In one of two patients with arterial postsphincterotomy bleeding, emergency surgery was required. Arterial bleeding from a gastric carcinoma induced by forceps biopsy stopped after intratumor application of fibrin sealant. This patient was electively operated after the routine staging procedure (Table 3).The overall mortality within 30 days was six out of 100 (6%). In four cases, deaths were closely related to the upper GI bleeding, whereas two patients died from a cardiac insufficiency and cerebral apoplexia, respectively. Local or systemic side effects due to the endoscopic application of the fibrin tissue adhesive were not observed.

Table 2. Overview of clinical results of endoscopic hemostasis by injection of fibrin sealant in 80 patients with peptic ulcer hemorrhage

	Stage of bleeding[a]				Total	
	Ia	Ib	IIa	IIb	*(n)*	(%)
Initial success of fibrin sealant	18/19	22/22	36/36	3/ 3	79/80	98.8
Recurrent bleeding	4/18	1/22	6/36	1/ 3	12/79	15.2
Definitive hemostasis	15/19	22/22	33/36	2/ 3	72/80	90.0
Surgery	4/19	0/22	3/36	1/ 3	8/80	10.0
Mortality (30 days)	1/19	1/22	3/36	0/22	5/80	6.25

[a] Categories according to the Forrest classification [5].

Table 3. Overview of clinical results of endoscopic hemostasis by injection of fibrin sealant in 20 patients with nonulcer hemorrhage in the upper gastrointestinal tract

	Initial success	Rebleeding	Definitive treatment	Mortality
Mallory-Weiss tear	6/6	0	–	0/6
Esophageal ulcer/esophagitis	5/5	0	–	0/5
Varices:				
Esophageal	0/1	–	Polidocanol	0/1
Fundic	0/1	–	Histoacryl	0/1
Duodenal	1/1	1/1	Histoacryl	0/1
Angiodysplasia	3/3	0	–	0/3
Sphincterotomy bleeding	2/2	1/2	Surgery	1/2
Gastric carcinoma	1/1	0	Surgery	0/1

Discussion

The results presented here clearly demonstrate that transendoscopic submucosal injection of a fibrin tissue sealant via a double lumen catheter is an efficacious and safe method to treat various bleeding lesions in the upper GI tract. We obtained fairly high rates of initial and definitive hemostasis in patients with nonvariceal bleeding. The data are in accordance with those reported by other authors [1, 4, 6, 8]. However, these encouraging results still have to be definitively confirmed by prospective, randomized, and controlled studies. A first attempt done by Strohm and coworkers in a small-scale randomized trial failed to demonstrate a statistically significant superiority of fibrin sealant over conventional sclerotherapy with adrenaline and polidocanol [9]. Therefore, the recommendation of a routine use of fibrin sealant for endoscopic sclerotherapy of bleeding lesions in the upper GI tract is presently based on the theoretical advantage of this physiological substance (avoidance of additional tissue damage, first step of wound healing), the results obtained in animal experiments in rats, and the experience of several investigators in large, but uncontrolled, studies.

Conclusions

Endoscopic submucosal injection of a fibrin tissue adhesive proved to be highly successful concerning initial and definitive control of upper GI bleeding predominantly due to peptic ulcers in an uncontrolled series of 100 patients. Local or systemic side effects were not observed. This clearly suggests fibrin sealant as a suitable substance for endoscopic sclerotherapy and as a highly valuable addition to the endotherapeutic armamentarium. However, before this therapeutic strategy can be recommended as the routine method of choice with any superiority compared to previous means of inducing hemostasis in GI bleeding, the results of further randomized and controlled studies have to be awaited.

References

1. Berg P, Born P, Barina W, Simon W, Zellmer R, Paul F (1990) Fibrinkleber versus Polidocanol bei der oberen Gastrointestinalblutung. Z Gastroenterol 28: 467
2. Chester JF, Hurley PR (1990) Gastric necrosis: a complication of endoscopic sclerosis for bleeding peptic ulcers. Endoscopy 22: 287
3. Cook DJ, Guyatt GH, Salena BJ, Laine LA (1992) Endoscopic therapy for acute nonvariceal upper gastrointestinal hemorrhage: a meta-analysis. Gastroenterology 102: 139–148
4. Eimiller A, Berg P, Bor P, Barina W, Paul F, Homann H (1989) A new development in gastrointestinal bleeding: sclerotherapy using a fibrin sealant. In: Waclawiczek HW (ed) Progress in fibrin sealing. Springer, Berlin Heidelberg New York, pp 131–134
5. Forrest JAM, Finlayson NDC, Shearmen DJC (1974) Endoscopy in gastrointestinal bleeding. Lancet II: 394–397
6. Friedrichs O (1992) Submucosal fibrin adhesion in peptic ulcer bleeding. Hellenic J Gastroenterol 5 [Suppl]: 86
7. Loperfido S, Patelli G, La Torre L (1990) Extensive necrosis of gastric mucosa following injection therapy of bleeding peptic ulcer. Endoscopy 22: 285–286
8. Salm R, Sontheimer J, Laaff H, Cegla M (1989) Tissue reaction and hemostatic characteristics – fibrin sealant versus polidocanol: experimental and clinical results. In: Waclawiczek HW (ed) Progress in fibrin sealing. Springer, Berlin Heidelberg New York, pp 123–129
9. Strohm WD, Römmele UE, Barton E, Weimer J (1992) Fibrinklebung und konventionelle Injektionstherapie bei blutenden Ulzera im oberen GI-Trakt. Z Gastroenterol 30: 687

Effects of Fibrin Sealant in Thyroid Surgery

M. Puccini, P. Iacconi, E. Ricci, and P. Miccoli

Abstract

During the last 6 months of 1991 we operated on 250 patients for thyroid diseases; among them, 116 were studied to evaluate the effects of a fibrin sealant (Tissucol, Immuno) in thyroid surgery. We analyzed our data with regard to the technique performed (total lobectomy, subtotal thyroidectomy, or total thyroidectomy), without considering basic illness. Patients treated with fibrin glue ($n = 51$) formed group 1. Untreated patients ($n = 65$) formed group 2.

Quantitative Analysis

Total Thyroidectomy (global data: group 1 ($n = 28$) mean = 82.39 cc (sd = 37.39). Group 2 ($n = 29$) mean = 121.79 cc (sd = 44.36). Single days: group 1: 72.18 cc (first day), 10.21 cc (second day). Group 2: 94.41 and 29.18 cc respectively. The difference between the groups is statistically significant ($p < .05$). The effect was observed using 1, 2 and 5 cc of Tissucol.

Subtotal Thyroidectomy (global data: group 1 ($n = 15$) mean = 75.8 cc (sd = 26.62). Group 2 ($n = 17$) mean = 160.59 cc (sd = 65.52). Single days: group 1: 69.72 cc (first day), 6.53 cc (second day). Group 2: 120.29 and 40.29 cc, respectively. The difference between the groups is statistically significant ($p < .05$). We observed the effect using 2, 2.5 and 5 cc of Tissucol.

Total Lobectomy (global data: ($n = 8$) mean = 51.25 cc (sd = 21.17). Group 2 ($n = 19$) mean = 86.32 cc (sd = 38.36). Single days: group 1: 45.87 cc (first day), 5.38 cc (second day). Group 2: 67.89 and 18.42 cc, respectively. The difference between the groups is statistically significant ($p < .05$). We observed the effect both using 1 and 2 cc of Tissucol.

Qualitative Analysis

- *Hematocrit:* A difference has been observed between the first and second postoperative days: group 1 from 8.8 % to 2 %; group 2 from 9.8 % to 6.9 %.
- *Red blood cells:* We observed a similar trend: group 1 from 839 270 to 210 000 RBC/mm^3; group 2 from 1 060 740 to 551 000.

- *White blood cells:* Group 1 from 8183 to 2063 WBC/mm^3; group 2 from 7168 to 10603.
- *Percentage of leukocytes:* No differences were observed between the groups.
- *Platelets:* In the first day we had a mean of 85000 in group 1 (sd = 24260) and of 129000 in the group 2 (sd = 23490).

Conclusions

The use of fibrin sealant (Tissucol, Immuno, Vienna) reduces surgical field bleeding in thyroid surgery, regardless of the surgical technique performed. The best results are obtained in subtotal thyroidectomy, a technique that, among those employed, leaves the largest bleeding surface; the results are scarcely influenced by basic illness. It permits a shortening of the postoperative period of hospitalization. The presence of fibrin glue determines a difference in the quality of secretion, too, indirectly reflecting its various effects on surgical wound.

Introduction

The application of fibrin glue on the surgical area at the end of an operation produces several effects thanks to its properties: the most evident is the reduction of serohematic secretions from the wound. At the beginning of 1991, we planned a study to evaluate this effect on the different surgical techniques performed for the treatment of thyroid diseases and to evaluate any possible modification in the composition of the fluid drained from the wound.

Material and Methods

During a period of 6 months (from July to December 1991) we operated on 250 patients affected by thyroid diseases. Patients submitted to the operation for the first time, unaffected by clotting or other hematological diseases, were informed about the study and asked to join it. A total of 116 gave their consent and were submitted to total lobectomy, subtotal thyroidectomy, or total thyroidectomy. The aim was to study the quantity of secretion drained off the surgical wound and its composition.

In some of the patients we applied fibrin glue (Tissucol, Immuno, Vienna) at the end of the operation, just before closing the anatomical layers, by means of mixing devices (Duploject, Immuno, Vienna) and nebulizing ones (Tissuspray, Immuno, Vienna) using oxygen as propeller, regulating its pressure by a proper set (Tissumat, Immuno, Vienna). The seal was prepared as suggested in the kit; we used a thrombin concentration of 500 IU/ml.

All patients had a continuous aspiration set (Redon-Flasche 400 cc., Mepra, Germany) and were submitted to short-term prophylaxis with a standard dose of antibiotic. The operations were performed by three surgeons, and the quantity of the fluid drained off the wound was measured by the personnel of the unit observing the graduated bottle. None of them knew whether the patient had entered the study or not. The fluid composition was analyzed by means of automatic counters in the hospital laboratory (Laboratory of Analysis, S. Chiara Hospital, Pisa): we sent a test-tube filled with fluid, asking for the hematocrit, number of red blood cells (RBC), number of white blood cells (WBC), and percentage of leukocytes.

We analyzed the quantitative data with regard to the techniques performed (lobectomy, subtotal thyroidectomy, or total thyroidectomy), each of them leaving a different bleeding surface.

A total of 51 patients were treated with fibrin glue and formed group 1; 65 patients were used as controls and formed group 2.

Data were processed by statistical analysis using descriptive statistics with Student's t-test for unpaired samples and Student's t-test for paired samples to analyze the changes in the fluid composition in a single group.

Results

Total Thyroidectomy

A total of 57 patients underwent total thyroidectomy, of which 28 were treated with Tissucol (group 1) and 29 formed the control group (group 2). The results of total secretion measurement (first plus second postoperative days) were 82.4 cc / 37.4 (mean / s.d.) in group 1 and 121.8 cc / 44.4 in group 2. The reduction of secretion in group 1 was statistically significant compared to group 2 (Student's t-test, $p < .05$; Table 1). This effect was observed using either 1, 2, 5 cc Tissucol (Table 2).

Table 1. Total thyroidectomy: total secretion

Group	Mean (cc)	S. D. (cc)	Range (cc)
1 (Tissucol, $n = 28$)	82.39	37.39	25–180
2 (Controls, $n = 29$)	121.79	44.36	40–230

S. D., standard deviation.

Table 2. Total thyroidectomy: effect of different amounts of Tissucol

Amount of Tissucol (cc)	Mean (cc)	S. D. (cc)	Range (cc)
1 ($n = 8$)	81.87	26.31	50–130
2 ($n = 13$)	95.00	44.95	25–180
5 ($n = 6$)	59.50	24.20	30– 90

S. D., standard deviation.

Table 3. Total thyroidectomy: daily section

Group	Mean daily secretion (cc)	
	1st p.o. day	2nd p.o. day
1 (Tissucol)	72.18	10.21
2 (Controls)	92.41	29.38

p.o., postoperative.

As regards group 1, the mean secretion was 72.2 cc during the first postoperative day and 10.2 cc during the second (Table 3). The corresponding values for group 2 were 92.4 cc and 29.4 cc, respectively. The hemostatic effect was already present on the first postoperative day.

Subtotal Thyroidectomy

A total of 32 patients were submitted to subtotal thyroidectomy. The mean total secretion in treated patients (group 1, $n = 15$) was 75.8 cc (s.d. = 26.6), while in control patients (group 2, $n = 17$) it was 160.6 cc (s.d. = 65.5). Also in this case the amount drained off was significantly lower in group 1 compared to group 2 ($p < .05$, Student's t-test; Table 4). The effect was observed using either 2, 2,5, or 5 cc Tissucol (Table 5).

In group 1 we measured 69.3 cc on the first postoperative day and 6.5 cc on the second. In group 2 the corresponding values were 120.3 cc and 40.3 cc, respectively. The hemostatic effect was already present on the first postoperative day (Table 6).

Table 4. Subtotal thyroidectomy: total secretion

Group	Mean (cc)	S.D. (cc)	Range (cc)
1 (Tissucol, $n = 15$)	75.80	26.62	40–115
2 (Controls, $n = 17$)	160.59	65.52	60–340

S.D., standard deviation.

Table 5. Subtotal thyroidectomy: effect of different amounts of Tissucol

Amount of Tissucol (u)	Mean (cc)	S.D. (cc)	Range (cc)
2 ($n = 8$)	81.87	25.63	40–110
2.5 ($n = 2$)	60.00	14.14	50– 70
5 ($n = 4$)	76.75	36.04	45–115

S.D., standard deviation.

Table 6. Subtotal thyroidectomy: daily secretion

Group	Mean daily secretion (cc)	
	1st p.o. day	2nd p.o. day
1 (Tissucol)	69.27	6.53
2 (Controls)	120.29	40.29

p.o., postoperative.

Total Lobectomy

A total of 27 patients were submitted to total lobectomy: eight from group 1 and 19 from group 2. The mean total secretion in group 1 was 51.2 cc (s.d. = 21.2) and 86.3 cc (s.d. = 38.4) in group 2. The mean quantity measured in group 1 was significantly lower compared to that of untreated patients ($p < .05$, Student's *t*-test; Table 7). The effect was observed using either 1 or 2 cc Tissucol (Table 8).

In treated patients, the mean quantity of secretion on the first postoperative day was 45.9 cc and on the second, 5.4 cc. The corresponding values for group 2 were 67.9 cc and 18.4 cc, respectively (Table 9).

As for the analysis of secretion patterns, we obtained a useful number of data, only for the first postoperative day. Few data were derived from the samples taken on the second postoperative day because of unexpected technical problems caused by the method employed (automatic counters). For this reason the mean values of the two groups referring to the second postoperative day were not compared; the time trend of the monitored parameters were evaluated only on the few paired samples we had (by Student's *t*-test for paired samples).

Table 7. Lobectomy: total secretion

Group	Mean (cc)	S.D. (cc)	Range (cc)
1 (Tissucol, $n = 8$)	51.25	21.17	20–80
2 (Controls, $n = 19$)	86.32	38.36	25–155

S.D., standard deviation.

Table 8. Lobectomy: effect of different amounts of Tissucol

Amount of Tissucol (cc)	Mean (cc)	S.D. (cc)	Range (cc)
1 ($n = 2$)	65.00	21.21	50–80
2 ($n = 6$)	46.67	20.90	20–80

S.D., standard deviation.

Table 9. Lobectomy: daily secretion

Group	Mean daily secretion (cc)	
	1st p.o. day	2nd p.o. day
1 (Tissucol)	45.87	5.38
2 (Controls)	67.89	18.42

p.o., postoperative.

Hematocrit

During the first postoperative day, we analyzed 94 samples, 42 from group 1 (mean value, 8.8%) and 52 from group 2 (mean value, 9.8%), which showed no significant difference.

During the second day, we received data referring to five samples from group 1 (mean, 2%) and nine from group 2 (mean, 6.9%). Despite these values, statistical analysis of the time trend did not reveal a significant decrease in either group (Table 10).

Red Blood Cells

During the first postoperative day we analyzed 102 samples: the mean number of RBC per volume unit was 873 270 in group 1 (data from 49 patients) and 1 067 740 in group 2 (data from 53 patients), with no statistically significant difference between them.

Six samples analyzed during the second postoperative day were from treated patients (mean, 210 000) and nine from untreated (mean, 551 000; Table 11). The statistical analysis for time trend showed a significant decrease in group 1 (Student's *t*-test, paired samples, $p < .01$), while the decrease was not significant in group 2.

Table 10. Hematocrit levels

Group	1st p.o. day mean/S. D. (%)	2nd p.o. day mean/S. D. (%)
1 (Tissucol)	8.79/5.22 (n = 42)	2.03/ 1.74 (n = 5)
2 (Controls)	9.75/7.44 (n = 52)	6.87/11.24 (n = 9)

S. D., standard deviation.

Table 11. Red blood cells

Group	No. of red blood cells/mm³	
	1st p.o. day	2nd p.o. day
1 (Tissucol)	893 270 (n = 49)	210 000 (n = 6)
2 (Controls)	1 060 740 (n = 53)	551 000 (n = 9)

p.o., postoperative.

White Blood Cells

We analyzed 103 samples during the first postoperative day. The number of WBC per volume unit was similar in treated (mean from 50 patients, 8183) and untreated patients (mean from 53 patients, 7168).

The corresponding values on the second postoperative day were 2063 (from six patients in group 1) and 10 603 (from eight patients in group 2), respectively (Table 12). Despite the difference showed by descriptive statistics, the statistical analysis of time trend revealed no significant variation in either of the two groups.

Percentage of Leukocytes

Data were obtained only from 18 patients regarding the percentage of leukocytes in samples, from group 1 and six from controls. The averages in the two groups were almost identical (Table 13).

Table 12. White blood cells

Group	No. of white blood cells/mm³	
	1st p.o. day mean/S. D.	2nd p.o. day mean/S. D.
1 (Tissucol)	8183/5099 (n = 50)	2 063/1 825 (n = 6)
2 (Controls)	7168/5812 (n = 53)	10 603/7 589 (n = 8)

p.o., postoperative; S. D., standard deviation.

Table 13. Percentage of leukocytes

Group	Neutrophils (%)	Lymphocytes (%)	Basophils (%)
1 (Tissucol, n = 12)	79.9	11.4	5.1
2 (Controls, n = 6)	79.5	11.7	5.9

Discussion

Human fibrin glue has several properties, which may be summarized as follows: tissue adhesion, hemostatic effect, stimulus to tissue regeneration, plastic effect, and anti-infective effect ([1, 2, 5, 6]; Tidrick and Warner, cited in [3]; Colvin, cited in [4]). It has been employed in man and its safety has been widely demonstrated [7]. In the treatment of thyroid pathology, it has been used both by echographists for conservative treatment of thyroidal cysts [8, 9] and by surgeons for thyroid surgery [10, 11]. Papers about surgery did not contain prospective studies, so we planned the present one so as to better evaluate the hemostatic effect of fibrin sealant in different surgical techniques and to examine whether the presence of glue induces any change in the composition of the fluid drained off the wound.

Our results show clear evidence of the hemostatic effect of the sealant employed. The effect is demonstrated in lobectomy, total thyroidectomy, and subtotal thyroidectomy, with a reduction in total secretions compared to controls of 41 %, 32 %, and 53 %, respectively. The best performance is obtained in subtotal thyroidectomy – which leaves the largest bleeding surface at the end of the operation – even using a moderate amount of Tissucol (2 cc). The hemostatic effect of fibrin glue is in general scarcely influenced by basic illness (nontoxic goiter, Graves' disease, thyroid cancer). The choice of the amount of sealant to apply should be based on certain aspects such as dimensions of the gland, basic illness, clotting system status, muscle cutting, and any other factor that could suggest major serohematic secretion.

The composition of fluids drained from both treated and untreated patients during the first postoperative day is almost the same, and the differences in mean values concerning the observed parameters between groups 1 and 2 is never of statistical significance.

The corresponding comparison between the groups during the second postoperative day has not been possible for the low number of relative data due to technical problems: only a few of the samples taken on the second day and sent to the laboratory were analyzed because of the small quantity of fluid, the presence of clots in the test-tubes, and several error messages given by the automatic counters. This caused us to consider only the time trend of the monitored parameters (hematocrit, RBC, WBC, and percentage of leukocytes) using a few paired data. This kind of analysis needs a different method to be fully carried out.

In our experience, the descriptive statistics show a decreasing trend of the hematocrit in both groups, being more evident in group 1, though not statistically significant. Also, the number of erythrocytes shows a tendency to decrease in both groups, statistically significant in group 1. These findings support our impression of a quicker change in secretion toward the serous phase in patients treated with fibrin glue. Maybe a new, complete study would give stronger evidence to support this impression.

The picture formed by descriptive statistics about WBC is interesting, too; it seems to suggest a decrease in the number of WBC as time passes in treated patients. The statistical analysis for time trend is not significant, but this is probably due to the limited number of observations. We interpret these data as the expression of other important properties of Tissucol: chemotaxis and non-specific immunity; in other words, we believe that many more leukocytes are trapped in the wound filled with fibrin seal. Several authors reported experimental and clinical evidence of chemotaxis and the antiseptic properties of fibronectin [4, 12–15] and of the tissue regeneration properties of thrombin and fibrin themselves [6, 12]. Thus, we think that a complete study could provide clinical evidence of this phenomenon, too.

Conclusions

The use of the fibrin sealant we tested (Tissucol, Immuno, Vienna) always reduces bleeding in thyroid surgery, regardless of the technique performed. In subtotal thyroidectomy, this effect allows a shortening of hospital stay, thus representing an economic advantage, too.

It generally affects hemostasis positively, acting on the final steps of the clotting system; we also believe that it influences the outcome, since it accelerates the healing process.

References

1. Pini Prato G P, Cortellini P, Clauser C, Guazzini S, (1983) Basi biologiche della sintesi tissutale con colla di fibrina humana. Min Stomat 32: 1–12
2. Donati L (1986) Indicazioni e limiti dell'uso della colla di fibrina (Tissucol) in chirurgia plastica. Proceedings of the XXXVth congress of SICPRE, Milano, 25–27 Sept 1986. In: Monduzzi (ed) Ia colla di fibrina (Tissucol) in chirurgia plastica. Milano, p 51
3. Frey M (1979) Die Vorteile der aufgeschobenen Spalthauttransplantation... Acta Chir Aust 11: 97–100
4. Schlag G (1988) Symposium on tisseel, 18 April 1988, Los Angeles, California, USA, pp 11–12 (abstract)
5. Harmand MF, Michel D, Bagot d'Arc M et al. (1986) Effect of fibrin seals on human fibroblast attachment and multiplication. European congress on biomaterials. Sept 1986, Bologna, Italy
6. Pohl J, Bruhn H D, Christophers E (1979) Thrombin and fibrin induced growth of fibroblasts: role in wound repair and thrombus organization. Klin Wochenschr 57: 273
7. Schlag G, Redl H (1986) General and abdominal surgery. Springer, Berlin Heidelberg New York (Fibrin sealant in operative medicine, vol 6)
8. Grandi M, Pederzoli S, Pradelli M et al. (1988) Proposta di una nuova metodica di trattamento medico della cisti tiroidea. Clin Ter 126: 329–334
9. Lobello R, Marranzini A, Cirillo M et al. (1989) Trattamento ecoguidato delle cisti tiroidee con colla di fibrina. Proceedings of the International Meeting "Eco Italia 89"
10. Peix J L (1988) Colle de fibrine et chirurgie thyroidienne. Lyon Chir 84(5): 384–385
11. Lombardi M, Giavazzi T, Mazzocchi G C et al. (1989) Particolari modalità d'impiego della colla di fibrina umana nella chirurgia tiroidea. Acta Chir Ital 45(3): 609–614

12. Kasai S, Kunimoto R, Nitta K (1983) Cross-linking of fibrin by activated factor XIII stimulated attachment, morphological changes, and proliferation of fibroblast. Biomed Res 4: 155
13. Fabrizio T, Nava M, Arioli N et al. (1990) Usefulness of fibrin glue in oncologic plastic surgery. Eur J Plast Surg 13: 201–205
14. Plow E F (1986) The contribution of leukocyte proteases to fibrinolysis. Blut 53: 1–9
15. Van der Ham A C, Kort W J, Weijma I M et al. (1992) Effect of antibiotics in fibrin sealant on healing colonic anastomoses in the rat. Br J Surg 79(6): 525–528

II. Pediatric Surgery

Fibrin Sealant in Paediatric Surgical Practice

V. Martinez Ibañez, A. Perez Martinez, and J. Boixochoa

Abstract

In 1987, we described the use of fibrin sealant for ensuring perfect haemostasis of the raw hepatic surface in reduced-size or partial paediatric liver transplantation. The success of our experimental and clinical studies led to new and wider surgical applications for this product. In liver transplantation, fibrin sealant was used to ensure high-pressure vascular anastomoses and to seal the raw surface in the reduced-sized liver. In these cases we sought efficacy in haemostasis, sealing and safety. The success of this high-risk surgery permitted us to employ fibrin sealant in other cases, including hepatic and splenic ruptures, complete tracheal stenosis treated with pericardial graft and thoracic and abdominal tumours, particularly bilateral Wilms' tumours, in which extensive tumourectomy must be performed in both kidneys and where the risk of urine and blood leakage is high. For all these indications the aim was the same: sealing. We have had no side effects or morbidity due to fibrin sealant. Thus, it was later applied in two cases of lymphangioma to avoid recurrence. At present, in rat models we are studying the possible use of fibrin sealant to prevent impending perforation provoked by neonatal necrotizing enterocolitis (NEC) and have applied it successfully in one clinical case. In this particular case, we used fibrin sealant by spray to avoid perforation and fixed the intestinal segments to prevent occlusive adhesions, and we used fibrin sealant without spray to apply a layer between the peripheral small intestine and the abdominal zip that was placed to control NEC evolution daily. It seems clear that new applications for fibrin sealant are emerging and our experience provides wider possibilities in paediatric surgery.

Introduction

When our paediatric liver transplantation (PLTx) programme began in 1985 [1], we were fully aware that the greatest limitation to the development of this procedure in children was the scarcity of paediatric donors. Thus, our goal was to study partial or reduced-size PLTx, which offers the opportunity of grafting adult donor livers into children. However, this feasible, but complicated surgical technique had one particular weakpoint: the hepatic raw surface after hepatectomy may produce haemorrhage and biliary leakage, the main factors of intra-operative haemorrhage or post-operative infections, which in turn may lead to morbidity and, on occasions, mortality.

As a consequence, our aim was to study different sealing substances in an attempt to avoid these kinds of complications.

Materials and Methods

Large-White pigs weighing between 10 and 15 kg were used as experimental animals. Orthotopic liver transplantations were performed [2].

Donor Operation

The animals were divided into two groups, A and B, each containing four subgroups. In all cases the donor liver was obtained, the gallbladder removed and the median lobe transected leaving as much raw surface as possible. The left lobe pedicle and left and middle hepatic veins are ligated. In group A, all vessels and biliary ducts in the raw surface were ligated, but in group B only the hiliar vascular structures and hepatic veins were ligated.

Following hepatectomy, different substances were applied: subgroup I (one animal), control with no substance; subgroup II (four animals), gelatin-resorcinol-formaldehyde glue; subgroup III (nine animals), Tissucol (Immuno, Vienna); subgroup IV (six animals), two layers of Tissucol with collagen felt inbetween.

Tissucol was applied by spraying with Duploject (Immuno, Vienna). Gas pressure was 1–2 bar for obtaining a gas flow of 5–10 l/min. A delicate, instantaneous fibrin film was formed. In group IV, collagen felt was cut and shaped to fit the raw surface and another layer of fibrin sealant applied.

Recipient Operation

A portojugular shunt was inserted and the recipient liver removed prior to orthotopic hepatic transplantation. No immunosuppressive therapy was given.

Results

We classified haemostasia in four degrees: Excellent (E), immediate haemostasia, no haemorrhage; good (G), minimal haemorrhage requiring additional sutures; deficient (D), significant haemorrhage which required other methods, and bad (B), uncontrolled haemorrhage.

The best results were obtained in subgroup IV (Tissucol and collagen), which was the only method with good haemostasis in group B (without ligatures). Results of subgroup III (Tissucol alone) were better than those of subgroup II (Table 1). Thus, the technique used in subgroup IV became our method of choice owing to its efficacy.

Table 1. Groups of study and results

	Group A (With ligatures)			Group B (Without ligatures)		
	n	H	Survival	*n*	H	Survival
Subgroup I	1	D	12 h			
Subgroup II	2	D	12/24 h	1	B	4 h
Subgroup III	4	E	7 days	1	B	6 h
		G	2 days			
		G	12 days			
		D	6 h			
Subgroup IV	2	E	4 days	4	E	9 days
		E	12 days		E	5 days
					G	1 day
					G	0 [a]

H, immediate haemostasia; E, excellent; G, good; D, deficient; B, bad.
[a] Death caused by air embolism.

In conclusion, the substance used in subgroup IV, i.e. fibrin sealant and collagen, has been our sealing substance of choice since we first performed reduced-size paediatric liver transplant [3, 4].

Discussion

The fact that both Tissucol and collagen are natural products and do not produce foreign body reaction or infection were added advantages, together with stimulated fibroplastic proliferation, collagen synthesis and wound healing. Both substances are biodegradable in vivo by plasminogen and collagenases present in inflammatory cells [5].

In addition, we also use Tissucol on vascular sutures (high-pressure anastomosis), portoenterostomy or choledoco-choledocostomy in all paediatric liver transplants. We observed no side effects or complications and therefore the field of application of Tissucol was widened to include surgical emergencies such as splenic and/or liver trauma.

Thus, we see that Tissucol is rapid, effective on haemostasia, seals with a high degree of cross-linking, is biocompatible, wound healing and safe with regard to transmission of viral hepatitis. All these advantages are applied in oncologic paediatric surgery in cases of thoracic surgery, particularly in axillary lymphangioma or thoracic neuroblastoma with dumb-bell-shaped elongation to a vertebral body or in abdominal surgery, e.g. in hepatic tumours [6], unilateral Wilms' tumour or in bilateral Wilms' tumour, where neoplasia has to be removed while preserving the kidney. Finally, we use it to prevent cervical lymphangioma recurrence.

The good results obtained with Tissucol in these fields encouraged us to test its usefulness in neonatology. Since 1989, for newborns with severe intestinal ischaemic lesions we have used an abdominal zip [7] to facilitate abdominal examination. Experience showed that the apposition of the plastic and intestinal layer could damage bowel tissue and provoke perforation, which could be avoided by a film of Tissucol inbetween. Consequently, we routinely use Tissucol on the intestine before closing the abdominal zip.

When we consider our experience with Tissucol and its consequences, we realise that we began with the most complicated cases, i. e. high-pressure anastomosis and hepatic raw surface; since then we have used Tissucol in many other less complicated, but always serious, situations, with good results. The journey was made backwards!

Acknowledgement. This work was supported in part by a 1986–1987 CIRIT Grant for Medical Research, Generalitat de Catalunya.

References

1. Martinez Ibañez V et al. (1985) Primeros trasplantes hepaticos infantiles en España. An Esp Pediatr 25: 477–480
2. Martinez Ibañez V et al. (1985) Nuevo modelo experimental de trasplante hepático en el cerdo. An Esp Pediatr 26: 107–110
3. Margarit C, Martinez Ibañez V, Lloret J et al. (1987) Segmental liver transplantation in pigs. Use of a fibrin sealant and collagen as haemostatic agents. Transplant Proc 19: 3835–3837
4. Margarit C, Martinez Ibañez V, Lloret J et al. (1988) Experimental and clinical reduced-sized orthotopic liver transplantation. Transplant Proc 20: 546–547
5. Schlag G, Redl H (1989) Fibrin sealant: efficacy, quality, and safety. In: Waclawiczek HE (ed) Progress in fibrin sealing. Springer, Berlin Heidelberg New York, pp 3–17
6. Martinez Ibañez V et al. (1989) Fibrin sealant in hepatic tumour surgery. Med Pediatr Oncol 17: 280
7. Martinez Ibañez V et al. (1992) "La cremallera abdominal" Una sorpresa quirúrgica. Cir Pediatr 5 (3): 182–183

Fibrin Sealant in Pediatric Surgery

K. Gdanietz and I. Gutsche

Abstract

After giving a brief historical survey of sealing procedures with biological sealant, we report our own experiences with Tisseel/Tissucol (Immuno, Vienna) in pediatric surgery. The use of fibrin sealant in neonatal surgery, especially for prevention of recurrent fistulas, on parenchymatous organs (birth injuries of spleen and liver), and on high-risk anastomoses in urology and septic surgery, is presented. It can be demonstrated that the use of fibrin sealant as quick and safe management is an advantage in pediatric surgery.

Introduction

In 1909, sealing procedures with biological materials were introduced. Fibrin began to raise interest as a physiological substance used for gluing tissue [1].

In 1940 Young and Medawar [19] used an adhesive fibrin substance obtained from chicken embryo extract as a biological glue. Following these first experiences, in 1944 Tidrick and Warner (cited in [10]) reported good clinical results achieved by the application of citrated plasma and thrombin in skin grafting.

In 1972 Matras et al. [11] were the first to use highly concentrated fibrinogen solution in combination with bovine thrombin solution to glue tissue. This marked the beginnings of the era of modern fibrin sealing [8]. In 1975 first reports on the clinical application of fibrin sealant were published by Sprängler [14]. Fibrin sealant was introduced in pediatric surgery in 1981 by sealing of a ruptured spleen [3]. Further reports were published on partial spleen resection [13], on the application of highly concentrated human fibrinogen [4] in 1982, and on fibrin sealing in congenital esophageal malformations [5]. The spectrum of indications has been gradually enlarged since then.

Material and Methods

For the use of Tisseel/Tissucol (Immuno, Vienna) in pediatric surgery, so-called absolute and optional (facultative) indications have been established on the

Table 1. The absolute indications for fibrin sealing in pediatric surgery

Esophagus
Atresia
Resection
Trachea/Lung
Tracheal resection
Segmental and lobe resection
Parenchymatous organs
Spleen:
Rupture
Partial resection
Envelopment after complete decapsulation by birth trauma
Capsula substitute
Liver:
Rupture
Resection
Covering the decapsulated liver
For reduced-size grafts in pediatric liver transplantation
Pancreas – traumatic lesion:
Resection
Pancreaticoenteroanastomosis
Maxillofacial surgery

Table 2. The relative (facultative) indications for fibrin sealing in pediatric surgery

Esophagus
Recurrent esophagotracheal fistula
Lung
Pleurodesis
Stopping air leakage
Parenchymatous organs
Abdomen:
Securing of anastomoses
Peritonization after retroperitoneal surgery
Prophylaxis of adhesions
Urology
Pyeloureteral anastomosis
Urethra-urethra anastomosis
Partial nephrectomy
Hypospadias
Epispadias
Orchidopexy
Plastic and reconstructive surgery
Skin transplantation
Bones
Cysts
Fixation of portions of articular cartilage
Septic surgery
Securing of intestinal anastomoses
Fibrin-antibiotic complex

basis of the personal experience of various authors and/or surgeons. The indications are summarized in Tables 1 and 2.

Thorax

Esophageal Atresia

Vogt [17] described four different types, with or without a communicating structure between the esophageal stumps and the tracheobronchial system. A special form is the so-called H-fistula.

Treatment of esophageal atresia aims at closure of the fistula and at establishing a continuous esophageal lumen. Previously, in order to prevent recurrence of the fistula, a muscle patch was interposed between esophagus and trachea. However, recurrence has not always been prevented in this way.

Instead of the muscle patch, we now use Tissucol, as demonstrated in Fig. 1. Morever, we apply the glue between the layers of the esophageal wall to be coapted, as described by Brands in 1983 [5]. Thus only four sutures between the upper and the lower part of the esophagus must be laid. The suture on the trachea is sealed, and the esophageal anastomosis embedded in fibrin sealant (Fig. 2).

Recurrent esophagotracheal fistulae can be closed endoscopically by means of Tisseel/Tissucol when they are not too broad. This technique was

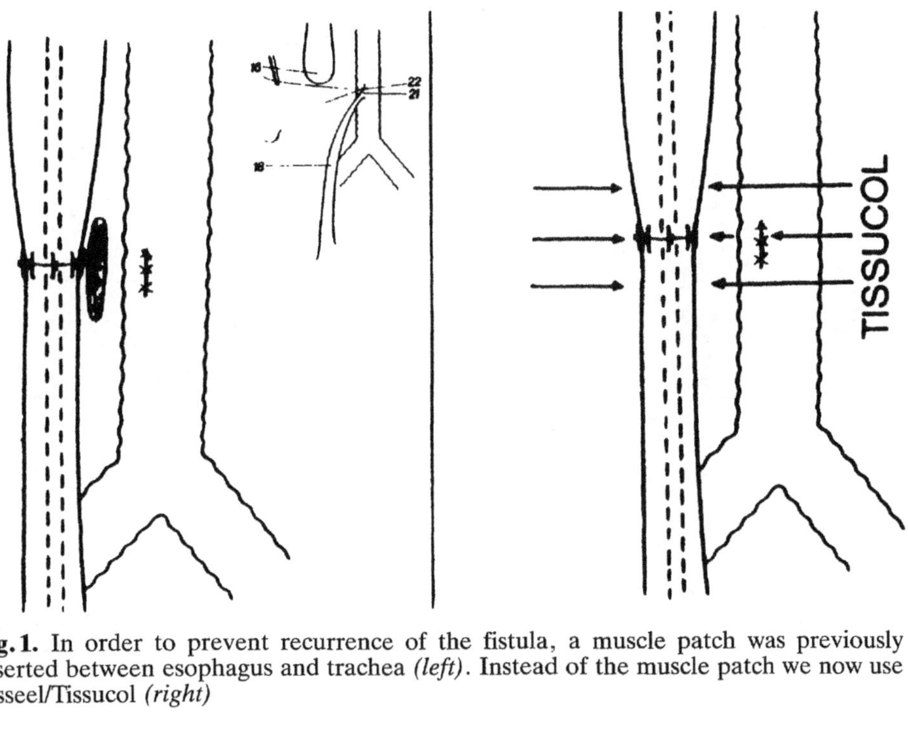

Fig. 1. In order to prevent recurrence of the fistula, a muscle patch was previously inserted between esophagus and trachea *(left)*. Instead of the muscle patch we now use Tisseel/Tissucol *(right)*

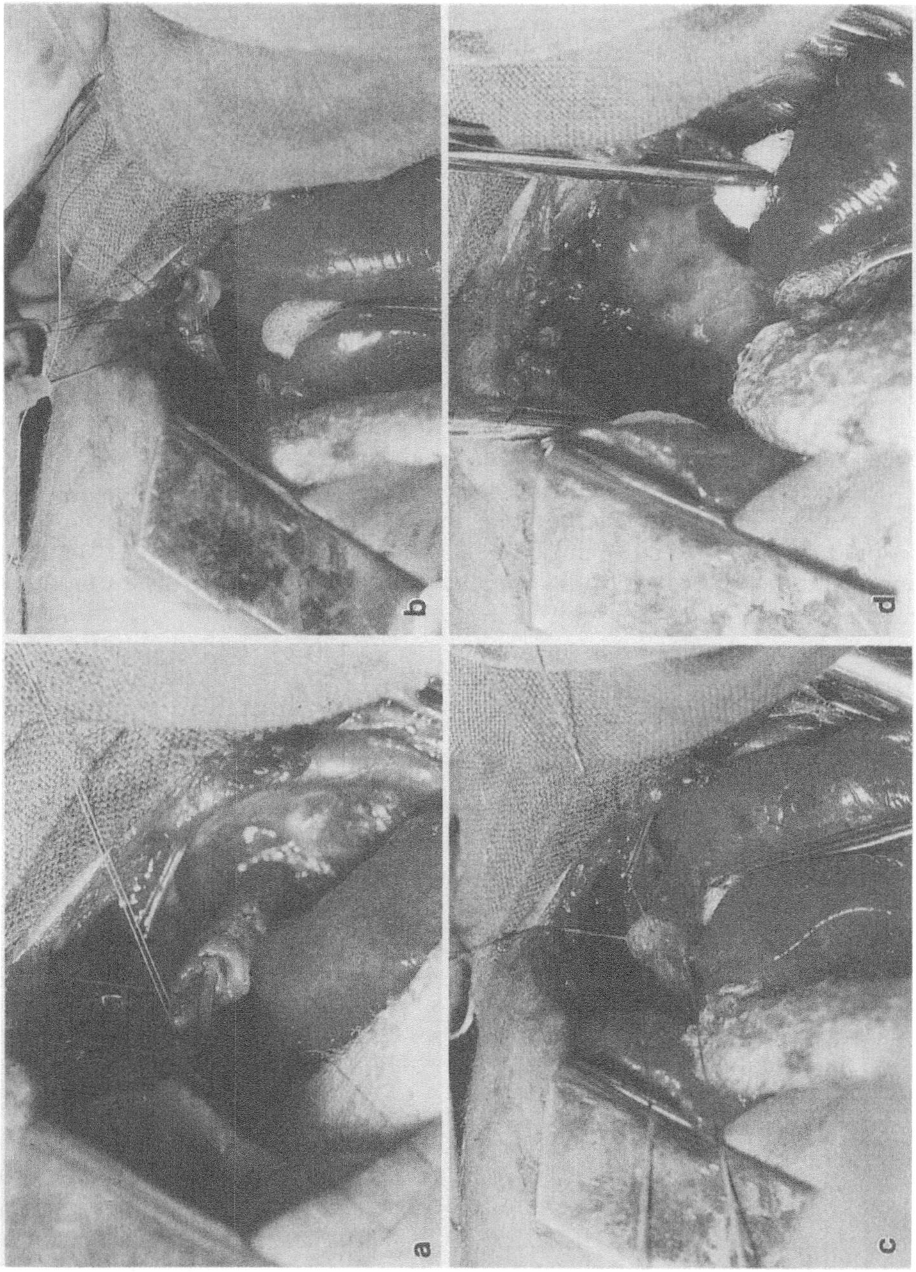

Fig. 2 a–d. Esophageal atresia, technique of the anastomosis using Tisseel/Tissucol. **a** After the segments have been freed sufficiently to permit them to be brought together with minimal tension, the anastomosis is started. **b** Applying the glue between the layers of the esophageal wall to be coapted. **c** The mucosal and muscular coats of the two segments are approximated with four interrupted 4–0 Vicryl sutures, between them the fibrin glue. **d** The esophageal anastomosis is embedded in fibrin sealant

Table 3. Endoscopical sealing for recurrence of esophagotracheal fistulas

Patient	Sex	Date of birth	Weight at birth (g)	Type of fistula	Age at gluing (days)	Glue	Outcome	Follow-up
1	F	26. 10. 72	2450	IIIb	255	Histoacryl	+	Healing
2	F	19. 11. 77	3600	IIIb	39	Histoacryl	+	Healing
3	F	3. 2. 79	3400	IIIb	190	Histoacryl	+	Healing
4	F	27. 10. 82	3100	IIIb	143	Fibrin sealant	+	Healing
5	M	8. 5. 84	2290	IIIb	25	Fibrin sealant (twice	0	Rethoracotomy, large fistula, died
6	F	1. 9. 84	2430	IIIb	53	Histoacryl	0	Rethoracotomy, chronic pulmonary patient
7	M	6. 12. 84	2590	III c	12	Histoacryl	0	Died after 12 days
8	M	20. 1. 85	3030	IIIb	44	Histoacryl, Fibrin sealant	0	Rethoracotomy, large fistula, healing
9	M	2. 6. 85	2700	IIIb	335	Histoacryl	0	Rethoracotomy, healing
10	M	4. 3. 86	3230	III c	46	Fibrin sealant	+	Healing
11	M	31. 3. 89	2140	IIIb	89	Fibrin sealant	+	Healing

F, female; M, male.

developed in our department and reported in 1974 [10]. Originally, we used Histoacryl (Braun-Melsungen).

After Tisseel/Tissucol became available we used this tissue adhesive. Eleven patients with recurrent esophagotracheal fistulae were endoscopically treated with different results (Table 3).

Details of endoscopic fibrin gluing of recurrent or congenital, isolated esophagotracheal fistulae have been published [7], referring to instruments, anesthesia, method of searching out the fistula, closure by gluing, and aftercare.

We use Tisseel/Tissucol after esophageal resection for stenosis ensuing from esophageal atresia repair. The anastomoses should be covered by fibrin sealant.

Trachea/Lung

In trachea and lung surgery, sealant is ideal to achieve hermetic sealing of the wound surface after tracheal resection and segmental and lobe resection. It successfully stops air leakage and can be used for pleurodesis. Spray application of fibrin sealant is suitable to guarantee a homogenous film of fibrin on the lung surface.

Abdomen

Fibrin sealant is generally applied to glue parenchymatous organs: spleen, liver, pancreas, kidney and lung. The following factors should be borne in mind when using fibrin sealant:

1. The application of fibrin sealant on the surface of resected organs stops blood or air leakage.
2. Fibrin sealing is most effective when the surface to be sealed is kept as dry as possible.
3. Two principles must be observed for the management of wound surfaces in parenchymatous organs:
   - Major blood vessels in the liver and of course biliary ducts should be ligated
   - Parenchymal wound surfaces of the spleen and liver should be covered with Tisseel-soaked fleece.
4. Securing of anastomoses by fibrin sealant is advantageous. The fibrin sealant covers the sutures and makes them immediately impermeable.
5. Tisseel/Tissucol allows an efficient peritonealization after retroperitoneal surgery (e.g., removal of tumors).
6. In abdominal organ resection and pediatric abdominal surgery, general abundant secretions are common because of the higher intercellular content of water in comparison with adults [2].
7. In most cases the use of fibrin sealant in abdominal pediatric surgery avoids postoperative draining (e.g., after peritonealization).

Splenic Surgery

Most experience has been gained with the spleen. Surgical interventions are aimed at organ preservation and the glue application is mostly combined with collagen fleece. In this organ, fibrin sealant is generally used in traumatic injury and helps to preserve this extremely important immune organ.

Rupture of the spleen in childhood is not always an indication for splenectomy. Roth and Daum recommend staging of the splenic rupture on a scale of I–IV, according to the surgical consequences in childhood [12].

One special case in neonate surgery is the treatment of a completely decapsulated spleen caused by birth injury. Upon laparotomy, a profuse quantity of blood gushed from the abdominal cavity. All splenic vessels passing through the hilus were immediately clamped. Since no material from the splenic capsula was available to cover the spleen, the entire organ was enveloped with fibrin (Fig. 3). A fibrin capsula substitute was formed and preserved the spleen. The patient's further course up to now, 3 years after operation, has been without complications [9].

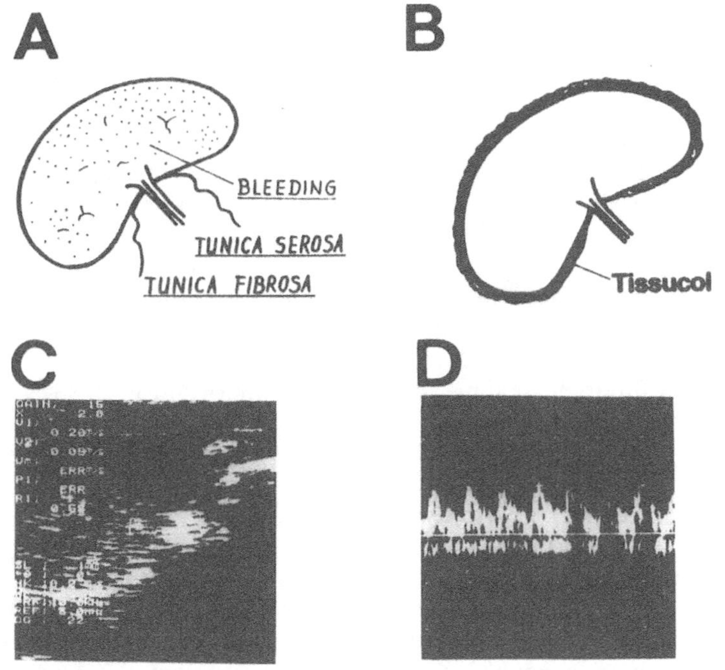

Fig. 3 A–D. Birth injury of the spleen. **A** Completely decapsulated spleen, the capsule had disintegrated. **B** The entire spleen enveloped in fibrin sealant. **C, D** Four months after operation, arterial blood flow is in the normal range for parenchymatous organs; normal blood flow in the splenic vein

Liver Surgery

In liver surgery, the tissue adhesive has proved extremely useful. Using it in combination with collagen fleece, the pediatric surgeon is able to close the liver surface after resection with reliability, provided that vessels and bile ducts have been ligated before. Also, decapsulated liver surfaces can reliably be covered by tissue glue, the anastomosis is complete, and a substitute capsule is formed. By means of fibrin glue and collagen fleece, we were able to stop bleeding from the left half of a liver decapsulated by birth trauma without problems. The use of fibrin sealant for reduced-size grafts in pediatric liver transplantation is reported. After meticulous hemostasis, the raw liver surface is covered with fibrin sealant and protected by an absorbable mesh. The procedure is performed ex vivo, keeping the liver immersed in ice-cold preservation solution except during application of the sealant.

In conclusion fibrin sealing guarantees a safe liver transplantation with reduced-size grafts [16].

Pancreatic Surgery

Possible indications for fibrin sealing in pancreatic surgery are traumatic lesions, resections of the head of the pancreas with pancreaticoenterostomy, reconstruction of the ductus pancreaticus, tail resection and left pancreatectomy, wedge excision, and enucleation.

The chief problem in pancreatic surgery is attaining hemostasis and fluidtight sealing of the secreting wound area. In this procedure, fibrin sealant is predominantly indicated, as it can significantly reduce the complication rate. In previous cases we used Histoacryl, but we now apply fibrin to the surface of the remaining pancreas and cover the sheets of the pancreaticodigestive anastomosis with Tisseel/Tissucol. In contrast to the usual procedure for the sealing technique, the sealant should not be applied in a thin layer but liberally. Hemostasis and fluidtight sealing are especially important in this region. We use no collagen fleece in pancreatic surgery.

Prophylaxis of Adhesions

To prevent recurrent intestinal obstructions, we no longer use Childs' and Phillips' technique of mesenteric plication. We perform sutureless plications with Tisseel/Tissucol. Therefore, all adhesions are dissected. The small gut is then arranged in equal loops and fixed by sealant. Lesions of the serosa can be sealed with fibrin glue.

On the basis of our experience, we are convinced that Tisseel/Tissucol is able to induce healing of serosal lesions and to prevent adhesions.

Septic Surgery

Fibrin sealant is known to stimulate the growth of fibroblasts and to attenuate the virulence of *Staphylococci* [1]. Animal experiments were carried out to examine the release of antibiotics from a fibrin antibiotic complex [18]. The fibrin antibiotic complex guarantees the maintenance of an effective antibiotic concentration for a short period of time. This technique can be used in bone infections [20]. In vitro comparative quantitative examinations concerning the growth of *Staphylococcus aureus* in solidified fibrin sealant and in blood clots have shown that in fibrin clots containing factor XIII, bacterial growth was reduced by more than 1 log step and in a factor XIII-free medium by more than 2 log steps.

Pathogenic germs (*Staphylococcus aureus*) grew much faster in blood clots than in fibrin clots; thus, it can be concluded that a fibrin clot does not entail a higher risk of infection than a blood clot.

In the case of incidental bacterial contamination, the growth conditions for the bacteria are significantly worse in a clot of fibrin sealant than in a blood clot. As compared to blood, fibrin sealant is a much less favorable culture medium for the growth of inoculated bacteria such as *Staphylococcus* and *Pseudomonas*.

Fibroblast stimulation and attentuation of the virulence of pathogens are advantages that can be exploited in infected wound areas. We are convinced that the following wound management was successful only on account of the use of fibrin intestine: a wide, infected, and entirely open wound area in the region of the lower abdomen, which was further complicated by the presence of a large intestinal fistula, was completely coated with fibrin sealant. The remaining portions of the abdominal wall were loosely fixed with sutures; three preceding operations had failed.

Urology

In our department we have used Tisseel/Tissucol in the following types of intervention:

- Ureteropelvic junction obstruction
- Reconstruction of the urethra (traumatic, bladder graft transplantation)
- Partial nephrectomy
- Hypospadias, epispadias
- Orchidopexy

In pediatric urology, the sealant is successfully applied in cases of hypospadias and epispadias. These operations are frequently followed by relapsing fistulae. Since the sealant is used for the firm joining of mobilized layers, the fistula rate has dropped considerably and hematomas are avoided. By application of Tisseel/Tissucol in surgery on renal parenchyma, safe hemostasis is achieved on large wound areas. The sealant can also be useful for the sealing of urethra-urethra and pyelo-uretero anastomoses.

Table 4. Use of fibrin sealant in pediatric surgery (1985–1992)

Type of surgery or indication	*n*
Abdominal surgery	
Esophagus and gastrointestinal tract	105
Liver	19
Spleen	18
Pancreas	1
Abdominal tumor	19
Urology	
Hypospadias	131
Bladder exstrophy	36
Ureteropelvic plastic surgery	35
Epispadias	5
Thoracic surgery	
Lobe resection	11
Segmental resection	21
Plastic surgery	
Graft transplantation	27
Other	
Struma resection	3
Bone cyst	13

Results

We have used Tissucol/Tisseel since 1985 (Table 4). Fibrin adhesive alone was enough to control bleeding in parenchymal organs. We were able to preserve a spleen which was totally decapsulated by birth trauma in a newborn. The spleen was embedded in fibrin sealant.

The glue can be used in lung surgery for sealing air leakages with good results. Since we have been using Tissucol/Tisseel in hypospadia repair, the rate of fistulas has rapidly dropped. We have seen no disadvantages using fibrin sealant.

Discussion

Fibrin sealant has brought considerable progress in pediatric surgery. Possible uses of Tisseel/Tissucol are surgical interventions in parenchymatous organs, the trachea, lung, and esophagus and in urology, plastic and reconstructive surgery, and septic surgery. Used in addition to conventional surgical procedures, there is less risk, especially in the resection of parenchymatous organs. A change has taken place in the operative procedure of esophageal atresia. After the tracheoesophageal fistula has been divided and the tracheal side is closed, the two segments are brought together by only four sutures if there is only minimal tension. We apply glue between the layers of the esophageal wall to be coapted, and in order to stabilize the anastomosis we embed this part in fibrin sealant. Previously, we made the anastomosis using a number of sutures.

To prevent recurrence of a fistula today, we use Tisseel/Tissucol instead of muscle patches between esophagus and trachea.

Fibrin sealant for hemostasis, e.g., on cut surfaces in spleen and liver and on completely decapsulated spleen and partial decapsulated liver by birth trauma, has proven to be effective, especially in combination with collagen fleece. In pancreatic surgery, we exceptionally apply a quantity of sealant to the cut surface without collagen fleece. In pediatric surgery, fibrin sealant in general can be used in all types of anastomoses: in esophageal surgery for the performance of hazardous anastomoses; in tracheobronchial surgery to seal air leakages; in pulmonary resection; and with gastrointestinal anastomoses, in which the glue covers the sutures and makes them immediately impermeable. However, not all pediatric surgeons use fibrin sealant for digestive anastomoses, because occlusion has been observed in some cases. We have not experienced complications from intraperitoneal application. Whether sealant provokes stenoses in ureteropelvic anastomosis after an Anderson-Hynes procedure needs further observation. On the other hand, we have had good experiences with fibrin glue in the reconstruction of the urethra (trauma).

Our results in treating hypospadias have been much better since we started using Tisseel/Tissucol, because we are able to join the mobilized layers firmly. In 80 cases no relapsing fistulae were seen.

Conclusions

The use of fibrin sealant in pediatric surgery results in definite advantages for both the surgeon and the child. It is a safe method for sealing cut surfaces of parenchymatous organs and for sealing high-risk anastomoses, because it reduces the rate of leaks. We feel that fibrin adhesive is also clearly indicated in septic surgery.

In view of our long-term results, we intend to carry on using Tisseel/Tissucol. It can be used in all areas of pediatric surgery.

References

1. Bergel S (1909) Über die Wirkung des Fibrins. Dtsch Med Wochenschr 35: 663–665
2. Becker C, Willital G (1992) Indication, technique and results of fibrin sealing in liver, pancreas, spleen and kidney resection in children. Report in "Update and future trends in fibrin sealing in surgical and non-surgical fields", abstract book paper no. 182, Congress Vienna/Austria, 15–18 Nov 1992
3. Brands W, Beck M, Raute-Kreinsen U (1981) Gewebeklebung der ruptierten Milz mit hochkonzentriertem Human-Fibrinogen. Z Kinderchir 32: 341–348
4. Brands W, Joppich I, Lochbühler H (1982) Anwendung von hochkonzentriertem Human-Fibrinogen in der Kinderchirurgie – ein neues Therapieprinzip. Z Kinderchir 35: 159–162
5. Brands W, Lochbühler H, Raute-Kreinsen U, Joppich I, Schaupp W, Menges H-W, Manegold BC (1983) Die Fibrinklebung angeborener Ösophagusmißbildungen. Zentralbl Chir 108: 803–807

6. Tidrick RT, Warner ED (1944) Fibrin fixation of skin transplants. Surgery 15: 90–95
7. Gdanietz K, Bunke K, Noack L. Ösophago-tracheale Rezidivfisteln und angeborene isolierte ösophago-tracheale Fisteln (H-Fistel). In: Technik der Fibrinklebung in der endoskopischen Chirurgie. Springer, (in press)
8. Gdanietz K, Gutsche I (1991) The use of fibrin sealant in pediatric surgery. Acta Chir Austriaca 3: 95–99
9. Gdanietz K, Gutsche I (1992) Notfallversorgung der Milz und Leber eines Neugeborenen mit Fibrinkleber. In: Gebhardt C (ed) Fibrinklebung in der Allgemein- und Unfallchirurgie, Orthopädie, Kinder- und Thoraxchirurgie. Springer, Berlin Heidelberg New York
10. Gdanietz K, Wiesner B, Krause I, Mau H, Jung fJ (1974) Gewebekleber zum Verschluß von Ösophago-tracheal-Fisteln bei Kindern. Z Erkr Atmungsorgane 141: 46–50
11. Matras H, Dinges HP, Lassmann H, Mamoli B (1972) Zur nahtlosen interfaszikulären Nerventransplantation im Tierexperiment. Wien Med Wochenschr 122: 517–523
12. Roth H, Daum R (1986) Fibrin sealing of parenchymal organs in pediatric surgery. In: Schlag G, Redl H (eds) General surgery and abdominal surgery. Springer, Berlin Heidelberg New York, pp 122–130 (Fibrin Sealant in operative medicine, vol 6).
13. Roth H, Daum R, Bolkenius M (1982) Partielle Milzresektion mit Fibrinklebung – eine Alternative zur Splenektomie und Autotransplantation, Z Kinderchir 35: 153–158
14. Sprängler HP, Holle J, Moritz E, Wolner E, Braun f, (1975) Experimentelle Untersuchungen und erste klinische Erfahrungen über die totale Blutstillung mittels hochkonzentriertem Fibrin. Österr Ges Chir 1975: 605–610
15. Seddon Hj, Medawar P (1942) Fibrin suture of human nerves. Lancet 11: 87–88
16. Ville de Goyet J, Hausleithner V, Reding R, Lerut J, Otte J (1992) Use of fibrin sealant for reduced size grafts in pediatric liver transplantation. Report in "Update and future trends in fibrin sealing in surgical and non-surgical fields", abstract book paper no 183, congress Vienna/Austria 15–18 Nov 1992
17. Vogt Eg (1929) Congenital esophageal atresia. Am J Roentgenol 22: 463–465
18. Wahlig H, Dingeldein E, Braun A, Kratzat R (1982) Fibrinklebung und Antibiotika-Untersuchungen zur Freisetzungskinetik. In: Cotta H, Braun A (eds) Fibrinkleber in der Orthopädie und Traumatologie vol 4. Heidelberger Orthopädie-Symposium, May 1981. Thieme, Stuttgart, pp 182–187
19. Young J, Medawar P (1940) Fibrin suture of peripheral nerves. Lancet 11: 126–129
20. Zilch H, Drehsen R, Lambris E, Hahn E (1982) Diffusionsverhalten von Cefotaxim aus der Fibrin-Antibiotika-Plombe im Tierversuch. In: Cotta H, Braun A (eds) Fibrinkleber in der Orthopädie und Traumatologie, vol 4. Heidelberger Orthopädie-Symposium, May 1981. Thieme, Stuttgart, pp 191–195

Indication, Technique and Results of Tissue Adhesive in Liver, Pancreas and Kidney Resection in Children

C. Becker and G. H. Willital

Abstract

We report our experience of tissue adhesive application in resection of the liver, the pancreas and the kidney in children. Different resection techniques using a laser, an ultrasound knife and diathermy for postoperative secretion, bleeding and infections is also reported. The different procedures are compared with each other with the additional use of tissue adhesives.

Introduction

Organ resections in children can lead to bleeding, infection and secretions. The success of resecting parts of the liver, the pancreas or the kidney depends very much upon excluding these post-operative complications, and different resection techniques can be used to avoid them. Since the possibility of using tissue adhesives became available, we have been able to close the surface of resected organs with high security.

The aim of this paper is to compare different resection techniques and to find out the advantages of tissue adhesives.

Material and Methods

We performed liver resections in 61 children, partial resections of the kidney in 29 children and resections of the pancreas in 54 children. The results concerning post-operative bleeding, secretions and infections are compared with a group of children treated with and without tissue adhesives. Regardless of the organ resected, the surface must be completely dry. Application of tissue adhesive has been performed using a double injection system, which makes it possible to achieve an optimal mixture of the two components fibrinogen and thrombin. Special care has to be taken in order to apply this tissue adhesive in a more or less homogenous fashion on the surface of the resected organs. In some cases, tissue adhesive was applied twice.

Table 1. Different pancreas resection techniques in children

	Haemostasis	Tissue closure	Pancreatic duct closure	Necrotic tissue (mm)
Co_2 laser	–	+	–	< 1
Nd:YAG laser	++	++	+	2–3
Cusa (ultrasound knife)	++	++	–	2–3
Diathermy	+	+	–	< 3

+, moderate; ++, high; –, none.

Different Resection Techniques in Pancreatic Surgery

Different resection techniques were evaluated and performed in pancreatic surgery in children using (a) diathermy, (b) ultrasound knife (Cusa technique; Cavitron, Stanford (A) and (c) laser (CO^2, neudynium: yttrium aluminium garnet, Nd:YAG)

These techniques have been evaluated with respect to post-operative bleeding, post-operative secretion, depth of local necrosis and closure of the pancreas ducts.

ND: YAG proved to be the best tool to achieve haemostasis. The pancreatic duct had to be closed in the normal surgical way in all cases. The area and the depth of local tissue necrosis is a little deeper using the ND:YAG laser compared to the CO_2 laser. With diathermy there were very frequently secretions and post-operative bleeding (Table 1).

Indication and Application of Tissue Adhesive for Abdominal Organ Resections

Liver Resections

Every liver resection must be performed with high security in order to prevent post-operative bleeding; especially in liver trauma and liver rupture, this is extremely important. The laser technique is the most adequate technique in this respect to perform organ-preserving resection. Using the laser in combination with fibrin application is the safest operative procedure to prevent post-operative secretion and post-operative bleeding. These two points were also important in preventing post-operative infections. The laser enables us to permanently close even very small vessels, regardless of whether they are part of the venous or the arterial system, and very small gall capillaries. In addition, the laser is very useful in children who had pre-operatively disturbances in blood clotting. Fibrin application in combination with the laser provides significant additional security for those areas where the laser application has possibly been performed inadequately. Laser application results in a completely dry area, thus creating an ideal surface for tissue adhesive therapy. The additional

Table 2. Liver resection techniques

Treatment	Secretion (ml)			Abscess	Gall secretion	Bloody secretion	Serous secretion
	Day 1	Day 2	Day 3	(*n*)	(*n*)	(*n*)	(*n*)
No tissue adhesive ($n = 20$)	112	75	42	5	6	7	7
Laser without tissue adhesive ($n = 22$)	54	30	20	6	3	5	14
Laser with tissue adhesive ($n = 19$)	55	15	10	0	1	3	15

application of collagen fleece is not necessary. Laser application made the collagen fleece superfluous (Table 2).

Kidney Resection

During the last 10 years partial resection of the kidney has been performed in 29 children. In kidney resections, small vessels belonging to the lymphatic system as well as small vessels belonging to the urinary system are cut and opened. Using the ND:YAG laser we were able to demonstrate by histological and electromicroscopical pictures that these connections and vessels can be closed completely. Cutting the organ using a scalpel or a sapphire knife opens up all these small vessels; there is a high frequency of tumor cell spreading using these techniques and using the diathermy, and the primary coagulation can be reopened by fibrinolysis later on [8]. Tissue adhesive was applied in combination with the laser in 12 children out of our series of 29 children (five who suffered from a kidney trauma, five children with a kidney tumour and two children suffering from a congenital kidney anomaly).

Post-operative complications, such as bleeding, infections and urinary fistulae, were significantly lower in those children treated with a combination of the laser and tissue adhesive application (Table 3) [6].

Table 3. Pancreas and kidney resection in children

	without tissue adhesive		with tissue adhesive	
	P	K	P	K
Bleeding	10/34	4/17	0/20	1/12
Infection	12/34	9/17	1/20	0/12
Fistulae	9/34	8/17	2/20	0/12

P, pancreas; K, kidney.

Pancreas Resection

Pancreas resections were necessary following pancreatic trauma, pancreatic tumours, pancreatic cysts and severe pancreatitis. Especially acute hemorrhagic pancreatitis is an indication to perform an urgent operation [3]. Pancreatic tumours in children are mostly adenomas necessitating a partial or subtotal pancreas resection [5, 7].

Pancreatic ruptures are primarily sequelae of abdominal trauma in children. The pancreas lying just in front of the vertebral column is compressed and sometimes ruptured completely in front of the vertebral column. In such an abdominal trauma, multiple organs sometimes have to be controlled for organ rupture, especially the liver and the spleen. We have to distinguish between four different degrees of pancreatic rupture (Fig. 1). Contusion of the pancreas leaves the pancreas capsule intact; these children can be treated conservatively, but the peripancreatic region has to be drained in order to avoid accumulation of pancreatic secretion in the retroperitoneal area. Subcapsular rupture of the pancreas leaves the pancreatic ducts intact and is treated by superficial sutures and tissue adhesives being applied on the surface of the pancreas. In cases of pancreatic rupture (complete or incomplete), a resection of this part is necessary. In these cases we use the laser resection technique in combination with fibrin sealing. The ultrasound technique (Cusa) enables us to separate pancreatic tissue. However, microruptures are caused in the whole area where the

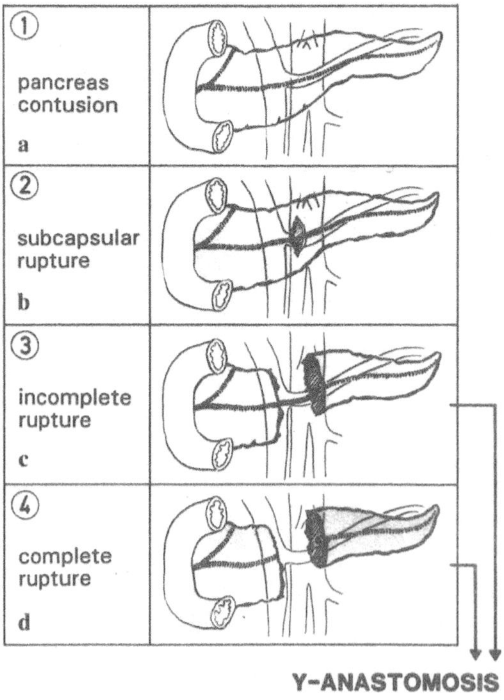

Fig. 1a–d. Survey of different types of pancreatic trauma in children. **a** Contusion of the pancreas. **b** Subcapsular rupture of the pancreas. **c** Incomplete rupture of the pancreas. **d** Complete rupture of the pancreas

ultrasound knife has been applied, leaving the tissue open. In pancreatic ruptures, the resection line is performed in an absolutely clean area and the Y-anastomosis of Roux is only indicated if a pancreas cyst is present. The application of fibrin or prolamin in the open pancreatic duct is not performed, because this occlusion is only temporary [2, 4]. The pancreatic duct is closed with a double ligature. The additional application of tissue adhesive gives the patient high security to prevent post-operative secretion at the resection line. As demonstrated in Table 3, this procedure has proved to be the safest one as far as post-operative infections, bleeding and secretion in pancreas resection are concerned (Fig. 1).

Discussion

The post-operative course depends very much on whether post-operative complications occur or can be avoided, i.e. bleeding, secretions and infections. Post-operative bleeding after liver or pancreas resections have a high mortality rate [1]. Post-operative infections lead to abscesses within the abdomen and organs and, furthermore, can lead to sepsis. Using the laser for organ resection, organs can be separated without any bleeding and without any secretion, thus creating an absolutely sterile surface. The additional use of a tissue adhesive with the laser provides the highest security rate.

References

1. Hollender L, Marrie A (1981) Chirurgische Behandlung der akuten Pankreatitis In: Allgöwer M, Harder F, Hollender LF, Peiper HJ, Siewert JR (eds) Chirurgische Gastroenterologie, Springer, Berlin Heidelberg New York, pp 1006–1011
2. Köckerling F, Zirngibl H, Gau FP (1992) Fibrinklebung in der Pancreaschirurgie. In: Gebhardt C (ed) Fibrinklebung. Springer, Berlin Heidelberg New York, pp 65–72
3. Kümmerle F, Neher M, Rückert K (1985) Pankreas. In: Kremer K, Kümmerle F, Kunz H, Nissen R, Schreiber HW (eds) Intra- und postoperative Zwischenfälle, vol 2: Abdomen. Thieme, Stuttgart, pp 135–161
4. Lorenz D, Wolff H, Waclawiczek H (1988) Die Pankreasgangocclusion in der Resektionsbehandlung der chronischen Pankreatitis und des Pancreaskopfcarcinomas. Chirurg 59: 90–95
5. Peiper HJ, Creutzfeldt W (1981) Endokrine Tumoren des Gastrointestinaltraktes. In: Allgöwer M, Harder F, Hollender LF, Peiper HJ, Siewert JR (eds) Chirurgische Gastroenterologie, Springer, Berlin Heidelberg New York, pp 585–600
6. Waclawiczek HH, Pimpl W (1986) Lymphfisteln nach Lymphknotendissektionen – Verhütung und Behandlung mit Hilfe der Fibrinklebung. Chirurg 57: 330–331
7. Willital GH (1992) Pancreasresektionen im Kindesalter mit Fibrinklebung – Indikationen, Resektionstechniken, Ergebnisse. In: Gebhardt C (ed) Fibrinklebung. Springer, Berlin Heidelberg New York, pp 217–226
8. Willital GH (1992) Nierenresektionen im Kindesalter mit Fibrinklebung – Indikationen, Resektionstechniken, Ergebnisse. In: Gebhardt C (ed) Fibrinklebung. Springer, Berlin Heidelberg New York, pp 227–232

Fibrin Sealing for Hemostasis of the Cut Surface in Reduced-Size Grafts During Orthotopic Liver Transplantation in Children

J. VALAYER, F. GAUTHIER, T. YANDZA, O. DEDREUZY, and A. LABABIDI

Abstract

Experience at the Pediatric Department of the Bicetre Hospital in Paris of liver transplantation in 105 children is reported, with special attention to reduced-size liver and related complications. Due to the young age of most patients, of which most were treated for biliary atresia, and the size discrepancy of the liver grafts usually retrieved from older donors and adults, a reduced-size liver graft was done in 59 % of the cases. Fibrin sealant was used to help with the control of blood oozing from the cut surface of the graft. However, a number of complications occurred, some of them in relation to the reduction of the graft size.

Introduction

During the last few years, there has been considerable development of liver transplantation in children, so much so that the demand for organs has increased well beyond the supply. Due to the scarcity of organs from brain-dead children, all transplant centers with a pediatric program are now familiar with reduced-size-liver (RSL) techniques, expanding the field livers can be harvested from to the much larger adult donor population [1]. We report our experience with RSL transplantation in children.

Materials and Methods

From January 1988 until October 1992, 105 children were treated by liver transplant in the Department of Pediatrics at the Bicetre Hospital, Paris. As in most pediatric programs, the majority of cases are *failures of Kasai's operation* for biliary atresia. A total of 20 retransplants were also done in this series, because of a number of complications dominated by hepatic artery thrombosis.

Mean age at operation was 3 years 5 months, with a mean weight of 13 kg. Thus, 58 % of transplantations were performed in children *less than 3* years of age. Mean age for children with biliary atresia was 2 years 1 month.

Generally, the donor to recipient weight ratio above which an RSL is necessary is just over 2, and in some cases a ratio as large as 10 or more has to be overcome. RSLs were used in all cases where donor to recipient body weight ratio exceeded 2, except for three cases where the donor weight was just above twice the recipient's.

Regarding age of recipient in relation to graft reduction, it appears that the younger the patient, the more need there is for reduction. It must be outlined, however, that we were reluctant to use very small livers from infant donors aged less than 6 months, because of the higher risk of hepatic artery thrombosis in these cases.

Liver was retrieved from brain-dead donors in all cases, in the course of a multiorgan procedure. Donor age ranged from 5 months to 47 years, with 46.7 % of them under the age of 10. During the year 1992, only 23 % of the donors were under 10, whereas the figure in 1988 was 77 %. Seven donors were aged 1 year or less.

Discrepancy in weight between donor and recipient was the reason for reduction of the graft in 59 % of cases (73 RSLs and 51 full-size livers, FSL). Reduction was a right hepatectomy or a right lobectomy, and in the latter the recipient's inferior vena cava was left in place in four instances. Only *one graft* resulted from a split liver, the right lobe transplanted to an adult recipient by another surgical team. Preparation of the graft, after reduction performed in University of Wisconsin cold-storage solution, was completed by routine application of fibrin sealant directly on the dried cut surface, a second application being sprayed over a collagen fleece tailored to the shape of the cut surface. The transplantation operation was performed following general procedural principles [2]. Particular technical problems related to pediatric transplantation and dealing with biliary atresia cases were encountered as in other series, such as tedious and hemorrhagic liver dissection following previous Kasai operation and development of portal hypertension, hypoplastic recipient portal vein to be bridged by anastomosis of the donor portal vein to the recipient superior mesenteric vein, and small hepatic recipient artery to be replaced by an iliac graft anastomosed to the infrarenal aorta. Differences in whole livers and RSL as regards operative data were significantly prolonged ischemia time, due to the 1–2 h extra needed for the reduction, but paradoxically nonsignificant higher amount of bleeding in the latter. In biliary atresia patients, however, both the tedious dissection of the native liver and the bleeding from the cut surface of the graft were cumulative reasons for significantly more severe bleeding, with the equivalent of nearly a mean of 4 whole blood volume units per child.

Results

The complications involved in liver transplantation are manifold. Taking in consideration only the *surgical complications*, it appears that a number of children are submitted to reoperation for different reasons, which may be vascular, biliary, or intestinal, not to mention retransplantation. *A total of 49 children were reoperated*, with a total number of 73 operations. RSLs were implicated in 44 reoperations, and FSLs in 29. Since so many factors contribute to the complications, no clear-cut correlation with reduction can be drawn from these figures; yet it should be underlined that with omission of the children that died during or soon after the transplant operation, *one child out of two* would have to be submitted to reoperation. Ten children were reoperated for control of *hemorrhage*, nine of which had RSL grafts. Two of these died in spite of reoperation.

Considering the rather specific pediatric complication of *hepatic artery thrombosis*, the 17 cases observed in this series were mainly due to small livers, with small arteries, the association small donor–small recipient being more prone to thrombosis. Reduction of the graft does not appear to have a protective role, since the figures are identical in both FSL and RSL, 13.7% and 13.6% of cases, respectively. The *mortality in this series is 17.1%*, a rather high figure due to a succession of recent complications which unfortunately occurred during the last year of the study in five children. Although there is a clear *predominance of RSLs* in the death cases (16 out of 18), the responsibility of RSL for mortality cannot be firmly established, since so many factors accumulate to create fatal complications.

The overall survival rate after transplant in this series is 82%. Of these 87 children with a follow-up of 1–58 months, the general condition is good for most, except for one awaiting retransplant and another with neurological complications. One year after transplantation, liver function is normal in 70% of cases, with immunosuppression by means of 5–20 mg cyclosporine/k per day and 0.5 mg prednisone/kg every 2 days. However, the long-term outcome of high blood urea and hypertension observed in 50% of cases will need further evaluation. No cases of lymphoproliferative diseases have yet occurred in this series.

Discussion

Among the number of complications following liver transplantation, intraoperative or immediate postoperative hemorrhage from the graft is the one to be feared most. All means of controlling the bleeding should be used. However, if it appears that the preparation of fibrin sealant (Tissucol, Immuno, Vienna) has unquestionable advantanges as regards control of blood and bileous oozing from capillaries and small bile ducts, it cannot be considered as a substitute for ligation even of small vessels encountered during the graft hepatectomy. We also found that adhesive strength resisted poorly to mobilization of the graft. As for complications related to the fibrin sealant, a case of an acquired antithrombin antibody was demonstrated when bovine thrombin was used, with no other manifestations than prolonged prothrombin time.

One question not related to the technique, but which is unavoidable and cannot yet be answered, is that of aging of a grafted liver retrieved from a donor in his forties or later, since maximum follow-up is only 8 years for the first RSLs.

In spite of the better access to organs created by the procedure of RSLs for children, the tremendous problem of the long period of time on waiting lists has not yet been completely solved. *The split liver technique* is another option, theoretically giving a chance to two patients instead of only one, the right part of the liver being used as a graft for another patient, yet it appears that there are some drawbacks to this technique. The logistic aspect of the operation is much more complicated if two teams are to be involved; also, complications are more prone to occur on both grafts, due to more delicate and distal preparation of vascular and biliary structures to be connected to the recipient's ones. Use of liver segments from a *living donor* has become a definite alternative to cadaveric graft retrieval in a number of selected centers throughout the world [3].

Our point of view is that the best graft is still a *FSL from a cadaveric pediatric donor* matching the recipient, with the exception of that from an infant donor exposed to hepatic artery thrombosis.

References

1. Otte JB, Ville de Goyet J, Sokal E, Alberti D, Moulin D, de Hemptinne B, Veyckemans F, van Obbergh L, Carlier M, Clapuyt P, Claus D, Jamart J (1990) Size reduction of the donor liver is a safe way to alleviate the shortage of size-matched organs in pediatric liver transplantation. Ann Surg 211: 146–157
2. Makowka L, Stieber AC, Sher L, Mieles L, Bowman J, Wallis Marsh J, Starzl T (1988) Surgical technique of orthotopic liver transplantation. Gastroenterol Clin North Am 17: 33–50
3. Broelsch CE, Whitington PF, Emond JC, Heffron TG, Thistlethwaite JR, Larry Stevens PD, Piper J, Whithington S, Lichtor JL (1991). Liver transplantation in children from living related donors. Surgical techniques and results. Ann Surg 214: 428–437

Changing Strategy in Splenic Surgery in Childhood

H. Roth, R. Daum, and Z. Zachariou

Abstract

Orthodoxly, splenectomy was the therapy of choice until the late seventies in splenic injuries. Thanks to increasing knowledge on the immunological importance of the spleen, especially in childhood, a change has taken place in the last decade, in favor of preserving splenic tissue or only monitoring the patient intensively when no life-threatening bleeding exists.

Due to modern technical methods such as fibrin sealing, it is possible to preserve splenic tissue. In our patients in the last 22 years, the strategy change can be clearly seen. Between 1970 and 1991, we treated 90 children with splenic rupture. From 1970 to 1980, 45 children out of 47 were splenectomized; however, from 1981 to 1991, only three out of 43 were splenectomized. All other patients were treated either conservatively or with tissue-saving operation methods using fibrin sealing.

Introduction

In previous decades, the idea that the spleen is not an indispensable organ and the lack of technical aids for operating on parenchymal organs dictated the procedure in splenic surgery. Splenectomy was the therapy of choice. Thanks to increasing knowledge on the immunological importance of the spleen in childhood [1, 4, 7, 8, 12–15] and to new operative techniques, a change has taken place in the past few years [2, 3, 9, 10]. Recently, even cases with splenic rupture and no life-threatening bleeding are treated conservatively under ultrasound and clinical monitoring [5, 16].

Technical Procedures for Saving Splenic Tissue

Surgical interventions in parenchymatous organs in children after injury are always aimed at organ preservation, repair, or tissue-saving resection. Due to the vulnerability of infantile tissue, surgical sutures are not always sufficient, even if atraumatic suture material is used. Laceration of the puncture channels and intersection of the parenchyma sometimes cannot be avoided, even if the knots are carefully dosed.

Modern coagulative techniques with infrared or laser radiation result in a more or less severe tissue necrosis, an undesirable side effect in pediatric surgery. Absorbable nets can contribute to compress the injured spleen, but the sole use of Vicryl (polyglactin 910) net or collagen fleece as a carrier for the blood coagulum does not guarantee safe hemostasis. Tissue sealants on the basis of cyanoacrylate are nowadays obsolete.

Using homologous absorbable fibrin sealant, especially in combination with collagen fleece, the pediatric surgeon now has a technique at his disposal that facilitates organ preservation and is a valuable complement or even alternative to sutures, partially avoiding additional loss of tissue. To summarize, surgical aids available for parenchymal organ operation include: (a) suture, (b) coagulation (infrared, laser), (c) Dexon (polyglycolic acid) net, (d) collagen fleece, and (e) glue (fibrin sealant).

Splenic Tissue Salvage Using Fibrin Sealing

The fibrin sealing system consists of two components: highly concentrated fibrinogen and the proteinase thrombin. It stimulates the last phase of the clotting cascade. As the two components in the presence of Ca ions combine during application, fibrin sealant consolidates, building a high degree of crosslinking due to factor XIII. Within 3–5 min, the fibrin net adhesions to the parenchyma are formed. Aprotinin is used as an antifibrinolytic agent.

The porous collagen has adhesive properties, with a special affinity to fibrin. The two components are simultaneously dripped onto the collagen fleece, which becomes humid and may be modelled like a capsule on the parenchyma.

The fibrin sealant and the collagen fleece are dissolved within the next few weeks or months due to phagocytosis and fibroblast activation, which results in rich soft tissue granulation. The predominance of transverse ruptures is due to the horizontal segmental situation of the vessels, which are functionally end arteries. In cases of partial splenic artery rupture, a sharp demarcation line sets the resection level. At this level, the parenchyma is dissected step by step and the surface of the remnant is sealed with fibrin and collagen fleece in a paving-stone manner (Fig. 1a). To assure safe sealing we put the collagen fleece over the capsule edge, thus creating a new capsule (Fig. 1b). Even the resection of a middle section is possible with this method when prehilus vascularization is present (Fig. 2). Atypical spleen segments can also be resected. Using fibrin sealant, deep sutures of the parenchyma can be omitted, saving more tissue that might otherwise have been destroyed due to reduction of vascularization.

Staging of Splenic Injury and Surgical Consequences

We recommend staging of the splenic rupture from I to IV stating the surgical consequences for each stage. Involvement of the splenic hilus and the clinical

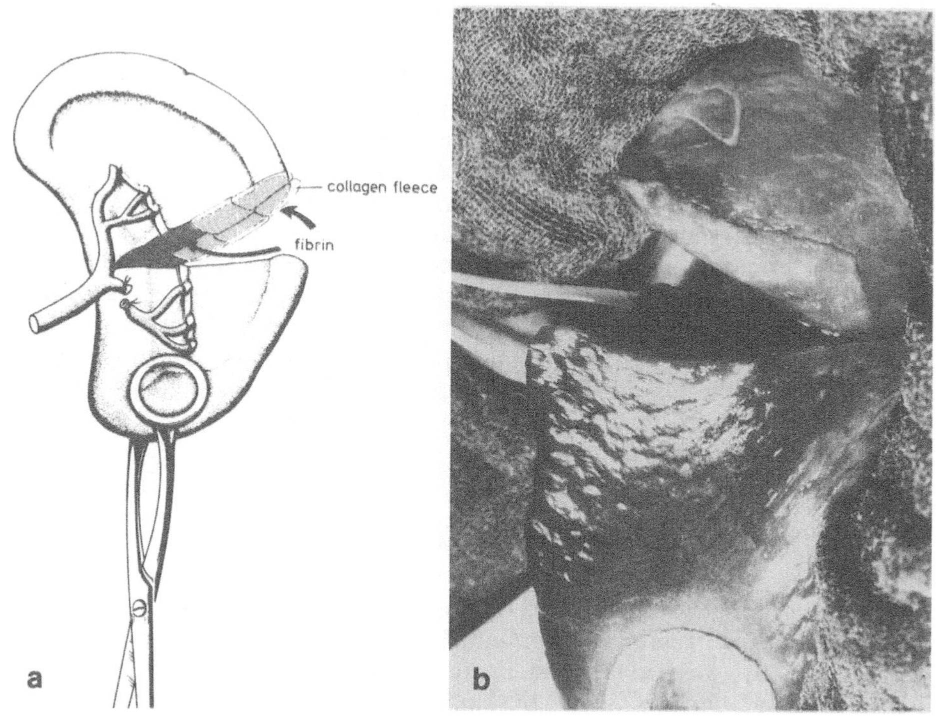

Fig. 1. **a** Hemisplenectomy using fibrin sealing and collagen fleece; **b** intraoperative situs of a splenic resection

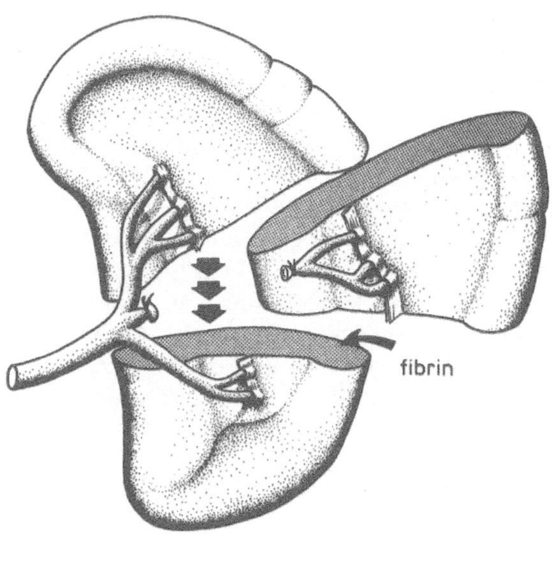

Fig. 2. Resection of a central segment

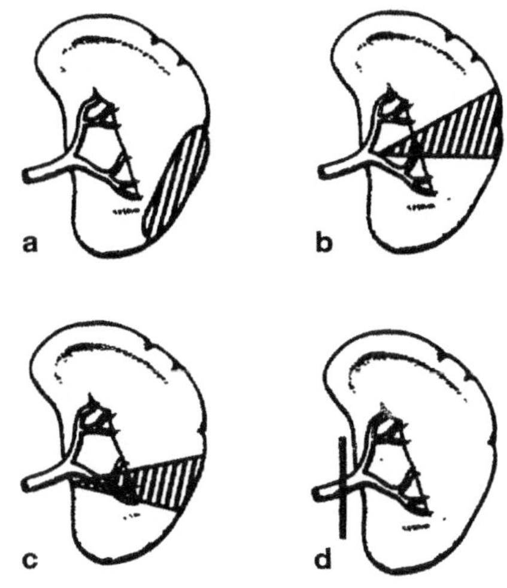

Fig. 3a–d. Staging of splenic injury and surgical consequences. **a** Stage I: peripheral rupture. Conservative treatment consists in intensive monitoring and operative treatment involves fibrin sealing.
b Stage II: rupture close to the hilus. Conservative treatment as for stage I; operative treatment involves suture of vessels and fibrin sealing. **c** Stage III: partial hilus injury, treated by segmental resection with fibrin sealing. **d** Stage IV: total hilus rupture, treated by subtotal resection or possibly autotransplantation

state of the child is decisive for management (Fig. 3). The predominance of transverse ruptures is due to the horizontal segmental situation of the vessels. Rare longitudinal ruptures are mainly outside the hilus area and can be managed easily. By peripheral ruptures we mean subcapsular hematomas and small lacerations of the parenchyma outside the hilus. We have two possible therapies at our disposal: (1) conservative therapy with supervision in an intensive care unit and (2) operative treatment by hemostatic parenchyma sealing. This treatment is seldom necessary, except in cases of multiple injuries of intra-abdominal organs where surgical intervention is necessary. Subcapsular hematomas are a classic example for conservative monitoring. In general, they can be well recognized by ultrasonography. Peripheral ruptures with considerable perisplenic bleeding should in no case be supervised outside a surgical unit if they are to be treated by conservative therapy. It is exclusively the decision of the surgeon whether he wants to perform a surgical intervention.

In contrast to former recommendations, ruptures close to the hilus do not necessarily need primary surgical treatment. Under the above-mentioned conditions of stable circulation and intensive monitoring, a "wait and see" attitude is justified. If an operation is performed, the spleen has to be mobilized from its ligamentous anchorage with ventral luxation.

In partial hilus injury, segment resection is the therapy of choice. In the presence of adequate vascularization, a middle segment can be excised and the remnant can be sealed with fibrin. There are two possible ways of managing a completely torn hilus: (1) subtotal resection and (2) autotransplantation of splenic tissue, a method propagated by many authors in recent years and questioned by others.

In cases of hilus rupture, preservation of the remaining spleen has absolute priority from the pediatric surgeon's point of view. This is almost always possible due to accessory vessels of the lower pole as well as the presence of a superior polar artery with maintenance of circulation of the remnant. Uncrit-

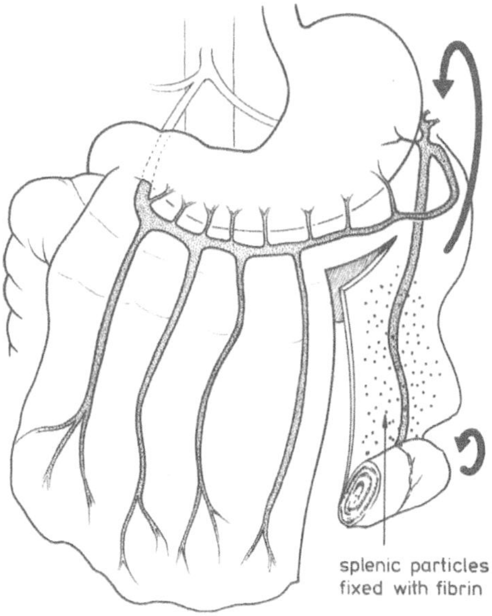

Fig. 4. Omentum flap formed for splenic autotransplantation and transferred to the splenic bed

ical application of methods described in the literature [11] is not only not useful, but dangerous as well, as the infant omentum is vulnerable. Our own experimental results show that autotransplantation of splenic tissue without fixation could result in ectopic splenic tissue and pseudoabscess. Only when there is close contact between the transplant and the omentum does neovascularisation occur in the form of a nidation. The fibrin spraying technique is a good method for fixation of splenic particles into the omentum. Another reason for not performing autotransplantation is that an adequate function of the transplantate is not present. In the rare case of autotransplantation in childhood, it should be performed into a left-pedicled omentum flap that is rolled up and transferred to the splenic bed so that misinterpretations of abdominal symptoms can be avoided (Fig. 4).

Changing the Operative Strategy

In our own patients of the last 22 years there has been a definite change in the therapeutic concept for splenic trauma. Between 1970 and 1991, we treated 90 children with splenic rupture. Looking at this time in two time periods, we can see the change: from 1970 to 1980, 45 children out of 47 (96%) were splenectomized and only two patients were treated with sutures (Fig. 5); however, from 1981 to 1991, 51% of the patients were treated with spleen-preserving methods, in 42% conservative therapy with monitoring was performed, and only in three cases was a splenectomy necessary (Fig. 6).

By analyzing splenic injuries according to stages I–IV, we can see that most of the patients in stage I and II were treated conservatively. The three splenec-

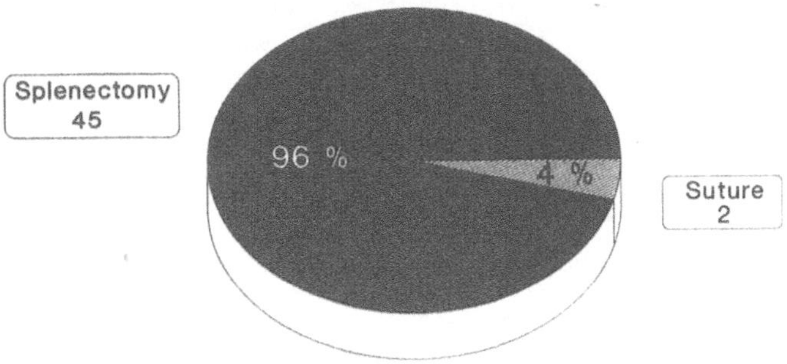

Fig. 5. Treatment of splenic rupture in Heidelberg from 1970 to 1980 (n = 47)

tomized children – stage II–IV – were treated before 1984, when the first steps for splenic salvage were made (Fig. 7). In the remaining 22 cases, 16 were stage II, five stage III, and one stage IV.

Conclusion

If surgical treatment is necessary after splenic rupture, fibrin sealing is in our experience the therapy of choice for splenic preservation. Regarding postsplenectomy complications, we agree with Morgenstern [6]: "the salvaged spleen or splenic remnant is a far greater trophy than the spleen in the pathologist's hand."

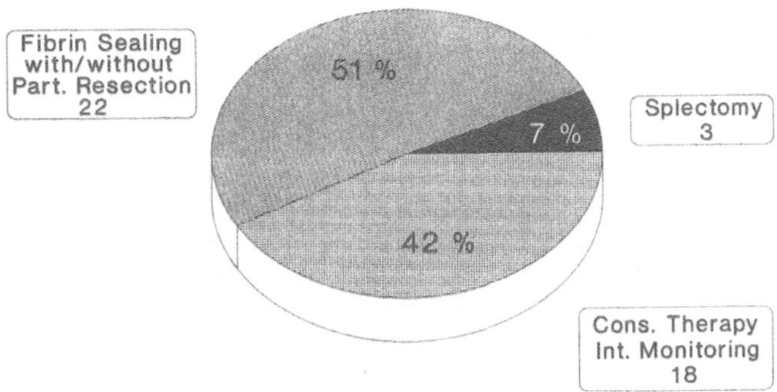

Fig. 6. Treatment of splenic rupture in Heidelberg from 1981 to 1991 (n = 43)

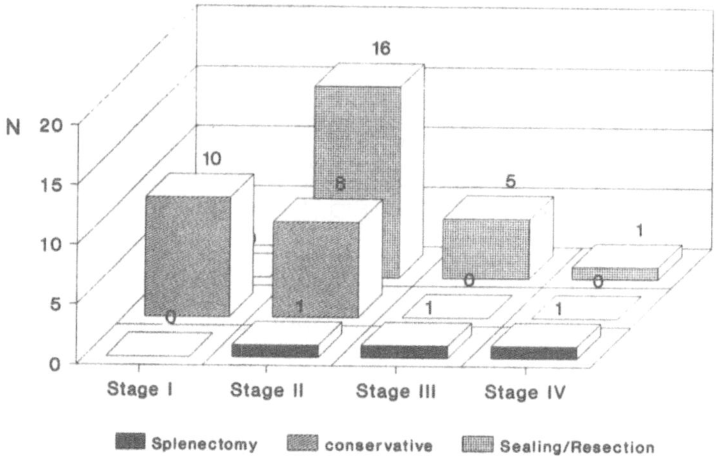

Fig. 7. Treatment of splenic rupture in childhood according to staging system (I–IV) in Heidelberg from 1981 to 1991 ($n = 43$). *Stage I*, peripheral rupture; *stage II*, rupture close to the hilus; *stage III*, partial hilus injury; *stage IV*, total hilus rupture

References

1. Balfanz JR, Nesbit ME Jr, Jarvis C (1976) Overwhelming sepsis following splenectomy for trauma. J Pediatr 88: 458–460
2. Buntain WL, Lynn HB (1979) Splenorrhaphy: changing concepts for the traumatized spleen. Surgery 86: 748–760
3. Burrington JD (1977) Surgical repair of the ruptured spleen in children. Arch Surg 112: 417–419
4. Ein SH, Shandling B, Simpson JS, Stephens CA, Bandi SK, Biggar WD, Freedmann MH (1977) The morbidity and mortality of splenectomy in childhood. Ann Surg 185: 307–310
5. Luna GK, Dellinger EP (1987) Nonoperative observation therapy for splenic injuries: A safe therapeutic option? Am J Surg 153: 462–468
6. Morgenstern L, Shapiro SJ (1979) Techniques of splenic conservation. Arch Surg 114: 449–454
7. Pedersen FK (1983) Postsplenectomy infections in Danish children splenectomized 1969–1978. Acta Pediatr Scand 72: 589–595
8. Roth H (1986) Infektionsrisiko und chirurgische Konsequenzen des Milzverlustes im Kindesalter. Langenbecks Arch Chir 369: 263–267
9. Roth H, Daum R, Bolkenius M (1982) Partielle Milzresektion mit Fibrinklebung – eine Alternative zur Splenektomie und Autotransplantation. Z Kinderchir 35: 153–158
10. Roth H, Daum R, Benz G (1986) Stadieneinteilung der Milzruptur – chirurgische Konsequenzen im Kindesalter. Chirurg 57: 194–197
11. Seufert RM (1983) Die Autotransplantation der Milz. In: Encke A, Kremer K, Ferdinand S (eds). Chirurgie der Milz. Hrsg. Enke, Stuttgart, pp 127–142
12. Singer DB (1973) Postsplenectomy sepsis. In: Rosenberg HS, Bolande RB (eds) Perspektives in pediatric pathology, vol 1, Year Book Medical Publishers, Chicago, pp 285–311
13. Wählby L (1981) Complications after elective splenectomy in children. Z Kinderchir 34: 56–60
14. Walker W (1976) Splenectomy in childhood: a review in England and Wales, 1960–1964. Br J Surg 63: 36–43

15. West KW, Grosfeld JL (1985) Postsplenectomy sepsis: historical background and current concepts. World J Surg 9: 477–483
16. Wiig JN, the Splenic Injury Study Group (1987) Splenic injury: a prospective multicentre study on non-operative and operative treatment. Br J Surg 74: 310–313

Management of Chronic Idiopathic Thrombocytopenia (Werlhof's Disease) by Partial Splenic Resection – An Alternative to Splenectomy in Childhood?

U. SPECHT, F. KIRCHMAIR, P. DEGENHARDT, H. MAU, and S. JAHN

Abstract

Medical management of chronic idiopathic thrombocytopenia (ITP) in childhood often fails [20, 26], which is why splenectomy is the recommended method of choice in these cases. However, surgery may not guarantee permanent therapeutic effects either: removal of the spleen may be accompanied by an increased risk of postsplenectomy infections (overwhelming postsplenectomy infection, OPSI syndrome). For these reasons we carried out partial splenic resection in nine children with chronic ITP. The aim of this procedure was to influence the course of chronic ITP by saving the immunological competence of children. Results from a clinical, hematological, and immunological point of view are discussed.

Introduction

Chronic idiopathic thrombocytopenia (ITP) is a rare autoimmune disease in childhood [12, 18, 19, 21]. In most cases, symptoms may be successfully influenced by corticosteroids, cytostatic treatment, or high-dose therapy with gamma globulins [4, 5, 11, 14, 22, 33], but it is also known, that permanent normalization of thrombocyte counts is not to be excepted right at the beginning of medical treatment for chronic ITP [13, 14, 24]. In only about 15 % of all pediatric patients with chronic ITP is a surgical intervention necessary. Following Katzenstein, in these cases splenectomy is the method of choice [6, 8]. Nevertheless, this approach fails in up to 20 %–30 % of children [15, 25, 28, 32] because of accessory spleens [6, 9, 15], persistent autoantibodies against platelets after splenectomy [23], or phagocytic activity of the mononuclear phagocytic system of the liver [15, 32]. In addition, the removal of the spleen, particularly during childhood, may result in a marked disturbance of immune balance accompanied by an enhanced risk of infection [7] and altered ontogeny of the immune system. Therefore, the decision for splenectomy in each particular case has to be made very carefully. It has to be pointed out that it is impossible to predict the effect of splenectomy on platelet counts or to make an individual prognosis of the course of ITP after operation. The success of splenectomy is probably a result of the removal of the spleen, which is considered to be the main place of pathogenic autoantibody formation and antibacterial antibody synthesis. However, regarding the risk associated with the removal of this immunologically important organ in childhood, partial splenectomy should result in a reduction of autoantibody production and probably a (temporary) beneficial clinical effect as well.

Patients

We first employed this technique in 1984, when we were asked by pediatricians to operate a child who had been treated with corticosteroids for chronic ITP for about 18 months, with remarkable side effects. This 7-year-old girl had undergone a partial splenectomy.

During the operation, we observed a macroscopically normal spleen, not enlarged, consisting of three segments. The spleen had been mobilized and the two ventral segments were removed. Our own operation technique is outlined in Fig. 1. Because the removal of splenic tissue had been done very intersegmentally, we did not observe any bleeding. To peritonealize the raw surface of the spleen, parts of the capsule were fixed with the help of fibrin glue (Tissucol,

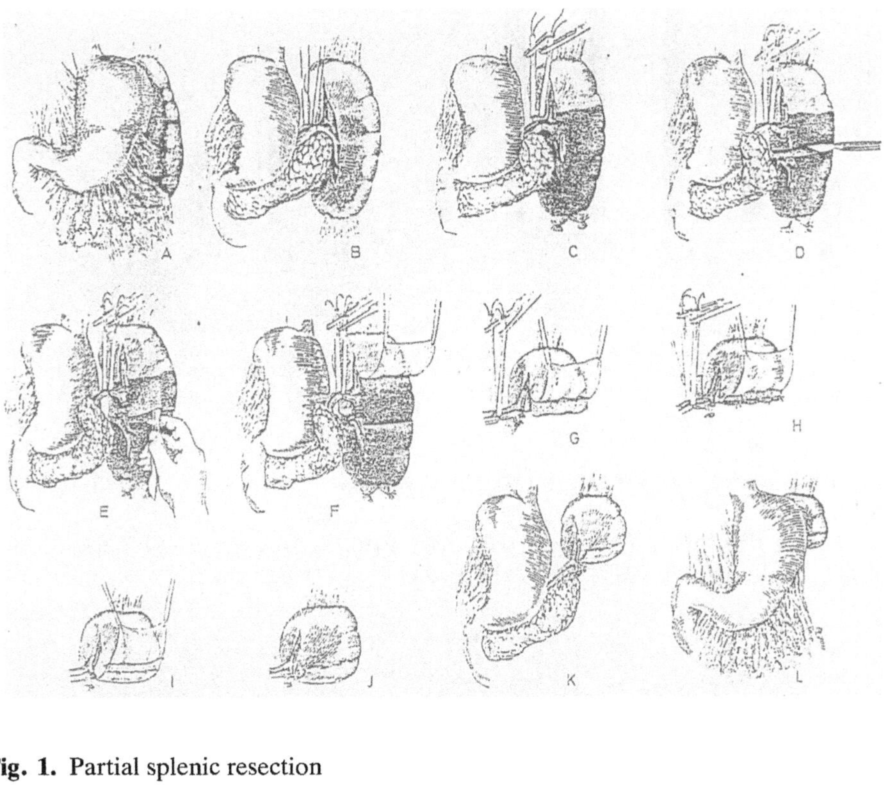

Fig. 1. Partial splenic resection

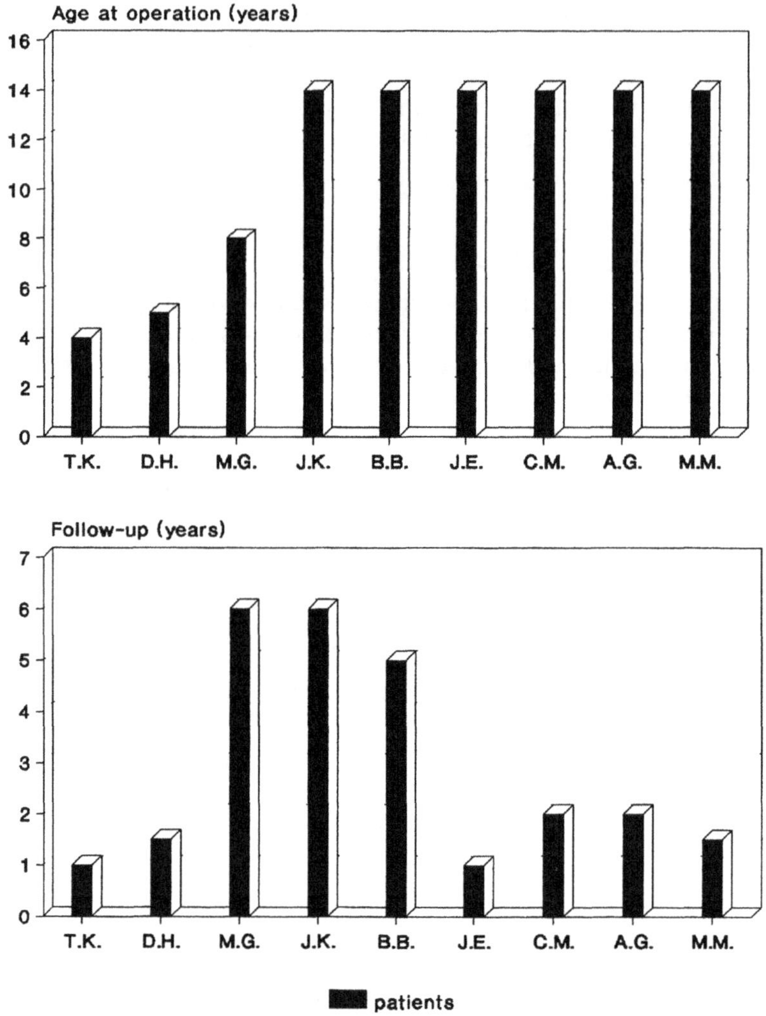

Fig. 2. Partial splenic resection in children suffering from chronic idiopathic thrombocytopenia (each *bar* represents one patient)

Immuno, Vienna). The retaining segment was nearly one third of the respective spleen mass.

During the following years, we carried out eight partial splenectomies in children with chronic ITP [30, 31] (Fig. 2).

Results

The results are presented in Fig. 3. We assessed platelet numbers and, parallel, analyzed the immune state and the yield of pitted erythrocytes. Furthermore,

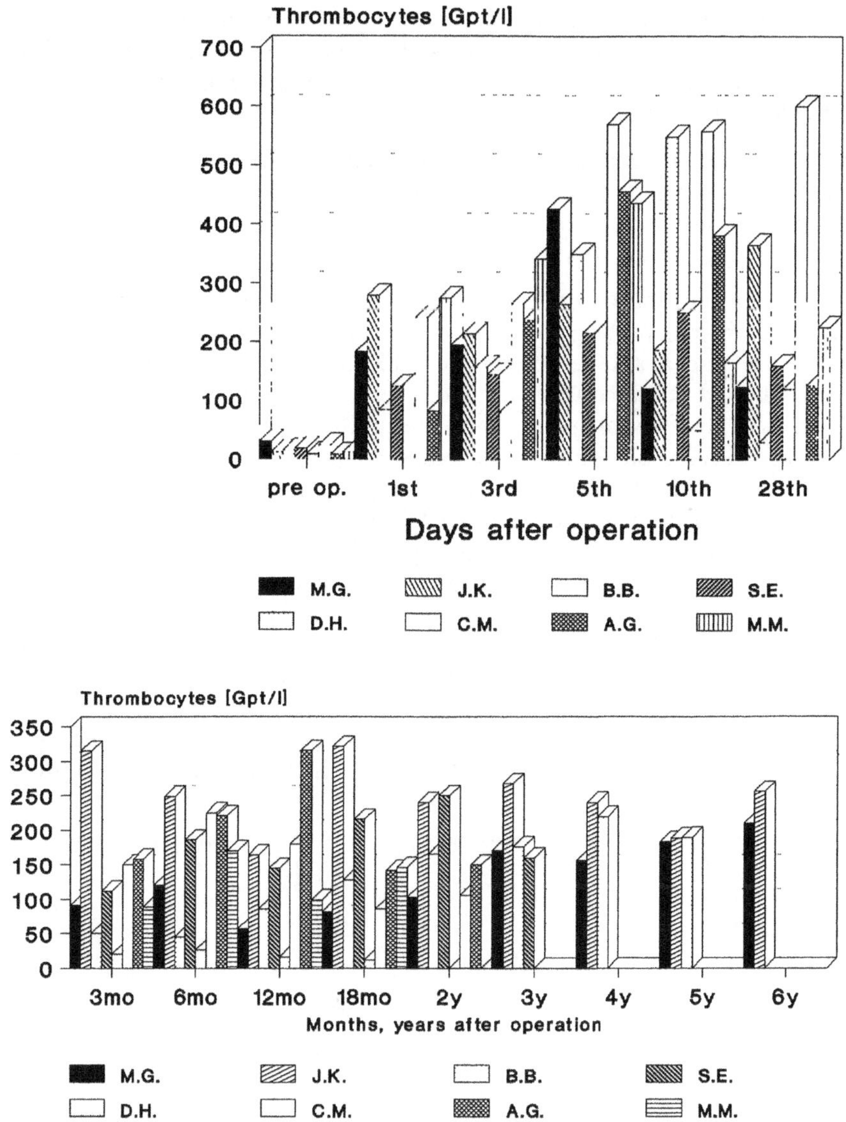

Fig. 3a, b. Development of thrombocyte counts in children with chronic idiopathic thrombocytopenia after partial splenic resection. *a* Early postoperative period; *b* late postoperative period (each *bar* represents one patient)

the retained spleen material was followed up functionally by Doppler ultrasonography and scintigraphy.

In each case, the partial splenectomy had a beneficial effect on thrombocyte counts immediately after the operation which lasted for the first 4 postoperative weeks. It should be mentioned however, that the postoperative time courses showed a very individual behavior, so that it is difficult to make any general conclusions. An interpretation of the operation results, in our experience, should be made after at least 12 months to obtain reproducible data.

Regarding the beneficial effect of partial splenectomy, patients can be divided into three groups:

1. Complete normalization of platelet counts (four patients)
2. Only partial remission of platelet counts, but significant clinical improvement (three patients)
3. Therapy failure (two patients)

In one case of therapy failure, however, a Fanconi-Zinsser syndrome was diagnosed, which is pathogenetically different from simple chronic ITP. For this disease, the partial splenectomy is most likely not an appropriate form of therapy.

The data obtained by immunological analyses may be of further interest. In each case, the partial splenectomy during the early postoperative time resulted in marked effects on lymphocyte subpopulation distribution, with a significantly reduction of the CD4 to CD8 ratio, also demonstrated by elevated numbers of HLA class II-positive (i.e. activated) T cells, mostly of the CD8-positive subclass. Moreover, the failure of B cells to produce human immunoglobulin G (IgG) following pokeweed mitogen stimulation in vitro has been detected. These data seem to be very similar to what is seen in splenectomized patients as long as 10 years after operation [17]. Serum levels of IgA, IgG and IgM, however, did not change.

In children with chronic ITP 22 months after partial splenectomy, we observed a normalization of pokeweed mitogen-induced IgG synthesis. In parallel, a significant reduction of the number of HLA class II T lymphocytes was seen (Fig. 4). Most importantly, just at the moment of improvement of

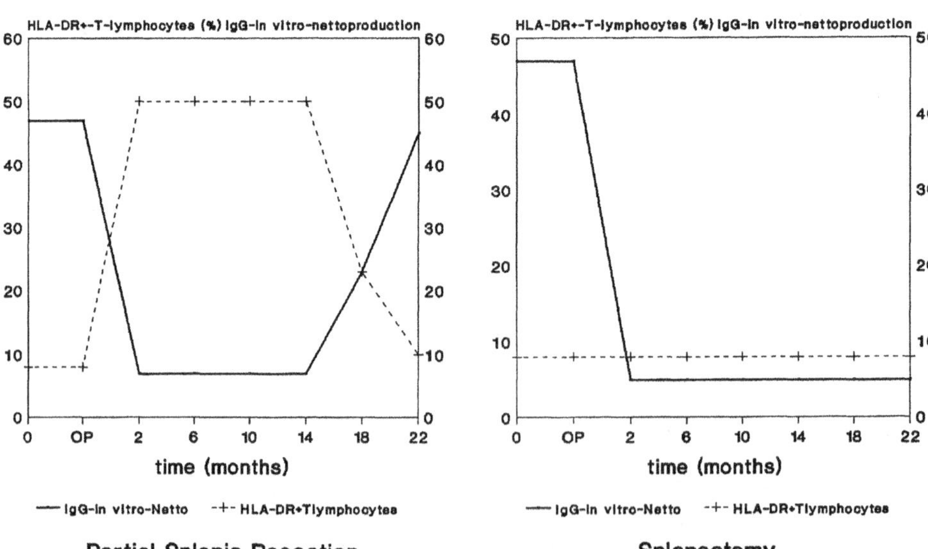

Fig. 4a, b. Time kinetics after partial splenic resection (*PSR; a*) or splenectomy *(b)* *Solid line*, in vitro immunoglobulin production after pokeweed mitogen stimulation. *Broken line*, percentage of HLA-DR T lymphocytes

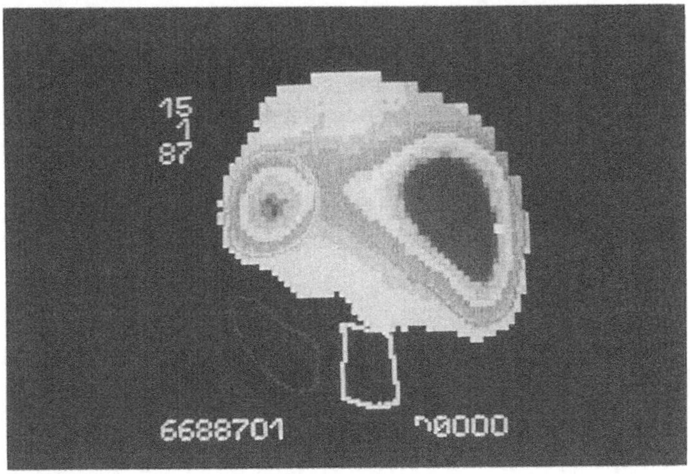

Fig. 5. Nuclide imaging demonstrates regular perfusion of the splenic remnant after partial splenic resection in a child with chronic idiopathic thrombocytopenia (splenic remnant on the *left* side)

immunological parameters, the number of thrombocytes rose, achieving nearly normal levels. In contrast to these data, a sufficient function of the spleen tissue was demonstrated in each patient (Fig. 5).

Discussion

Chronic ITP is an autoimmune disease characterized by the occurrence of IgG autoantibodies binding the gp IIb–IIIa membrane glycoprotein complex on platelets [3, 10, 16, 23, 28]; the percentage of children developing a really chronic process is quite low [21, 27, 28].

However, most children show symptoms of ITP in connection with bacterial and viral infections. The rate of spontaneous remission is probably higher than usually expected from data obtained from adults [1, 2.]. The hypothesis was suggested that this may be explained, at least in part, by a higher reconstitutional capacity of the immune system in childhood. During recent years, the spleen has been considered to be the main place of autoantibody production. Our recent data regarding the treatment of chronic ITP by partial splenectomy support this hypothesis and, furthermore, raise the following more or less hypothetical points: in previous studies, we pointed out that every surgical treatment of the spleen influences the immune state [17, 30, 31]. In this context it should be mentioned that the consequences of partial versus total splenectomy for the time course of the immune parameters are quite different [17]. Partial splenectomy results in immunological alterations of a transient character, which may be improved by mechanisms which until recently were unknown. The manipulation of the spleen obviously generates a disturbance of the immune system in infants and children due to altered regulatory processes.

Our own studies on the determination of serum autoantibodies against platelets in a few cases ruled out that partial splenectomy resulted in a significant decrease of such immunoglobulins.

Further studies must be carried out to give a definitive statement on our hypothesis that partial splenectomy in childhood may have a curative effect on autoantibody production.

Unfortunately, we are not able to give a definitive answer at present as to whether partial splenectomy is an alternative method to cure chronic ITP in childhood.

References

1. Andrew M, Blanchette VS, Adams M, Ali K, Barnard D, Chan KW, de Veber LB, Esseltine D, Israels S, Korbrinsky N (1992) A multicenter study of the treatment of childhood chronic idiopathic thrombocytopenic purpura with anti-D. J Pediatr 120: 522–527
2. Bellucci S, Bordessoule D, Coiffier B, Tabah I (1989) Interferon alpha-2b therapy in adult chronic thrombocytopenic purpura. Br J Haematol 73: 578–579
3. Bizzaro N (1992) Familial association of autoimmune thrombocytopenia and hyperthyroidism. Am J Hematol 39: 294–298
4. Blanchette VS, Kirby MA, Turner C (1992) Role of intravenous immunoglobulin G in autoimmune hematologic disorders. Semin Hematol 29[Suppl 2]: 72–82
5. Boughton BJ (1991) Anti-D Ig for treatment of immune thrombocytopenic purpura [letter]. Blood 78: 2157–2158
6. Buchanan GR (1989) Overview of ITP treatment modalities in children. Blut 59: 96–104
7. Cario W.-R, Mau H, Specht U, Zimmermann HB (1986) Vermeidbarkeit des OPSI-Syndroms. Pediatr Grenzgeb 25: 239–249
8. Cohen MA, Bourstyn E, Galera MJ, Najean Y, Clot P (1991) Splenectomy for chronic thrombocytopenic purpura. Ann Chir 45: 540–542
9. Dan K, Gomi S, Kuramoto A, Maekawa T, Nomura T (1992) A multicenter prospective study on the treatment of chronic idiopathic thrombocytopenic purpura. Int J Hematol 55: 287–292
10. De Souza SJ, Sabbaga J, d'Amico E, Pasqualini R, Brentani R (1992) Antiplatelet autoantibodies from ITP patients recognize an epitope in GP IIb/IIIa deduced by complementary hydropathy. Immunology 75: 17–22
11. Feliu E (1992) The treatment of idiopathic thrombocytopenic purpura (ITP) or Werlhof's disease. An Med Intern 9: 108–111
12. Fujimura K, Kuramoto A (1991) Physiopathology and therapy of idiopathic thrombocytopenic purpura. J Jpn Soc Intern Med 80: 855–859
13. Giers G, Salama A, Mueller-Eckhardt C (1992) Rhesus (D)-IgG-antibodies in the treatment of autoimmune thrombocytopenia. Dtsch Med Wochenschr 117: 1–5
14. Gorski J, Czestochowska E, Tyminski W, Kicinska M (1989) Use of vincristine-loaded blood platelets, danazol and gamma globulin in the treatment of patients with idiopathic thrombocytopenic purpura. Acta Haematol Pol 20: 65–71
15. Harwood SJ, Carroll RG (1992) Functional studies of left upper quadrant mass aid management of idiopathic thrombocytopenic purpura. Clin Nucl Med 17: 652–655
16. Imbach P, Tani P, Berchtold W, Blanchette V, Burek-Kozlowska A, Gerber H, Jacobs P, Newland A, Turner C, Wood L (1991) Different forms of chronic childhood thrombocytopenic purpura defined by antiplatelet autoantibodies. J Pediatr 118: 535–539
17. Jahn S, Specht U, Neuhaus K, Haensel K, Volk H.-D. (1987) Unterschiede im Immunstatus bei Kindern nach Splenektomie bzw. Milzteilresektion. Z Klin Med 42: 1137–1140

18. Kiefel V, Santoso S, Kaufmann E, Mueller-Eckhardt C, (1991) Autoantibodies against platelet glycoprotein Ib/IX: a frequent finding in autoimmune thrombocytopenic purpura. Br J Haematol 79: 256–262
19. Koyanagi H, Kishida K, Shimomura K, Kurokawa M, Deguchi T, Shimoda Y (1992) Immunological study of childhood acute ITP at onset. Pediatr Hematol Oncol 9: 11–19
20. Kuriya S, Nomura T (1989) Prognosis of chronic thrombocytopenic purpura. Acta Haematol Jpn 52: 1379–1385
21. Lilleyman JS (1984) Idiopathic thrombocytopenic purpura – where do we stand? Arch Dis Child 59: 701–703
22. Mizutani H, Furubayashi T, Imai Y, Kashiwagi H, Honda S, Take H, Kurata Y, Yonezawa T, Tarui S, Ikehara S (1992) Mechanisms of corticosteroid action in immune thrombocytopenic purpura (ITP): experimental studies using ITP-prone mice, (NZW × BXSB) Fl. Blood 79: 942–947
23. Mizutani H, Furubayashi T, Kashiwagi H, Honda S, Take H, Kurata Y, Yonezawa T, Tarui S, Ikehara S (1992) Effects of splenectomy on immune thrombocytopenic purpura in (NZW × BXSB) Fl mice: analyses of platelet kinetics and antiplatelet antibody production. Thromb Haemost 67: 563–566
24. Mori PG (1991) Thrombocytopenia: therapeutic aspects in the child. Haematologica 76 [Suppl 3]: 131–137
25. Podolak-Dawidziak M, Kuliszkiewicz-Janus M, Kielan W, Werynska B, Niewolna M (1989) Circulating immune complexes in chronic thrombocytopenic purpura in adults before and after splenectomy. Pol Arch Med Wewn 82: 175–183
26. Poliakov VE (1991) Idiopathic thrombocytopenic purpura (Werlhof's disease) in children. Feldsher I Akusherka 56: 25–28
27. Robb LG, Tiedeman K (1990) Idiopathic thrombocytopenic purpura: predictors of chronic disease. Arch Dis Child 65: 502–506
28. Smith NA, Boughton B (1992) More on anti-D for the treatment of splenectomized patients with immune thrombocytopenic purpura [letter]. Blood 79: 1891
29. Smith NA, Chakraverty RK, Obeid D, Boughton BJ (1989) Long-term response in a patient with ITP following low dose anti-D immunoglobulin therapy. Autoimmunity 4: 115–117
30. Specht U, Mau H, Winter H, Jahn S, Klemp E (1988) Ergebnisse und postoperative Milzfunktion nach Milzteilresektion wegen chronisch-idiopathischer Thrombozytopenie. Kongreßberichte zum 17. Hämophilie-Symposium. Springer, Berlin Heidelberg New York
31. Specht U, Mau H, Winter H, Jahn S, Volk H-D, Cario W-R (1988) Partial splenectomy for treatment of chronic idiopathic thrombocytopenia in childhood. Folia Haematol 115: 509–514
32. Tomer A, Hanson SR, Harker LA (1991) Autologous platelet kinetics in patients with severe thrombocytopenia: discrimination between disorders of production and destruction. J Lab Clin Med 118: 546–554
33. Vermylen C, Bugnon F, Ninane J, Cornu G (1990) Treatment of immune thrombocytopaenic purpura in childhood. A review of 146 patients. Acta Clin Belg 45: 120–125

Fibrin Sealing in Pediatric Esophageal Surgery

V. Jasonni, P. E. Caffarena, G. Martucciello, G. Mattioli, and P. L. Lelli Chiesa

Abstract

Fibrin sealing is of great importance in the surgical treatment of the most important esophageal malformations and other conditions affecting children.

Between 1984 and 1992 we operated on 84 patients with esophageal atresia using direct anastomosis, six patients with atresia using esophagocoloplasty, and one patient with a rare acquired tracheoesophageal fistula, one patient with esophageal duplication, and three patients with severe stenosis following caustic esophagitis using end-to-end esophageal anastomosis. In all 95 patients, fibrin sealant (Tissucol, Immuno, Vienna) was used in order to consolidate the sutures. None of our patients showed surgical complications or problems caused by the use of fibrin sealant. In our experience, its main advantage consists in consolidating sutures and reducing the risk of anastomotic leaks.

Introduction

Esophageal surgery in children presents serious problems in the treatment of malformations, in which it is necessary to restore esophageal continuity either with direct end-to-end anastomosis or with the interposition of intestinal segments [4, 9].

In patients with esophageal long-gap atresia and especially in the case of a direct anastomosis, the final suture can be characterized by a certain tension. Analogous situations occur, for example, when end-to-end anastomosis is performed in patients with stenosis following caustic esophagitis [8].

In pediatric surgery, the use of fibrin glue [1] for the consolidation and sealing of esophageal anastomoses is not as diffuse as in other branches of general surgery. The authors report their experience in the use of this plasma derivative in esophageal atresia, acquired stenosis, and other rare esophageal malformations occurring in childhood.

Materials and Methods

We used industrial preparations [8] now available consisting of a lyophilized plasma derivative composed of fibrinogen and factor XIII (Tissucol, Immuno, Vienna). These preparations play an important role in the process of coagulation, since, together with calcium chloride-activated thrombin, they determine fibrin production. Fibrin binds to the cell membrane and adheres firmly to tissue, thus starting the initial phase of wound cicatrization. Moreover, an enzyme inhibitor, aprotinin, is added to fibrin and factor XIII. The function of aprotinin is to slow down fibrinolysis, which is a normal occurrence in wound healing. The time taken by fibrin sealant to solidify is proportionate to the concentration of thrombin and calcium chloride added to the lyophilized component and to the time of contact.

The mechanism of action is similar to the classical coagulation process. Factor XIII is activated by calcium chloride and thrombin and, by acting on fibrinogen, it determines fibrin polymerization. The result of this process is the rapid formation of an insoluble fibrin clot. At the same time, plasmin, which determines the subsequent clot resorption, is blocked by aprotinin.

This preparation was used from 1984 to 1992 in 239 operated children; 95 of them, aged between 1 day and 13 years, were affected by esophageal malformations and can be classified as follows: 84 cases of esophageal anastomosis and six cases of esophagocoloplasty because of esophageal atresia; one case of esophageal duplication; three cases of end to end esophageal anastomosis because of acquired caustic stenosis and one case because of closure of acquired esophageal fistula.

In 89.3 % patients with esophageal atresia, direct anastomosis was performed at neonatal age (type III atresia); in 10.7 % of patients (nine affected by type I atresia), surgery was delayed, since the distance at birth between the two esophageal pouches did not allow us to perform anastomosis in the neonatal period (Table 1).

Table 1. Delayed Anastomosis (atresia type I without fistula)

Patient number	Sex	Age at hospitalization	Gap at operation	Age at operation (months)
1	m	Newborn	2	3
2	m	1 month	4	3
3	f	6 months	3	6
4	m	Newborn	2	4
5	m	Newborn	2	3
6	m	6 months	1	6
7	f	1 month	2	3
8	m	2 months	3	4
9	m	Newborn	3	3

m, male; f, female.

In each patient, an average quantity of 5–10 cc of fibrin sealant was applied on the suture rima using the Duploject system (Immuno, Vienna).

Results

In 78 % of our 95 operated patients, different degrees of suture tension were present, especially in cases of long-gap atresia. After surgery, fibrin glue application made it possible to obtain an immediate consolidation and sealing of the suture. Only in one case was a partial leak of the anastomosis observed, requiring conservative treatment with total parenteral nutrition and thoracic drainage.

Gastroesophageal reflux was present in 25 % of esophageal atresia. All the patients had normal esophageal canalization allowing oral feeding (Fig. 1).

Postoperative endoscopic calibrations of the esophagus were necessary in all cases of delayed anastomosis.

Discussion and Conclusions

The results obtained demonstrate that a correct surgical approach [5, 6] in the treatment of esophageal malformations in childhood, associated with the use of fibrin glue, can considerably reduce postoperative complications.

In our series, it was possible to restore esophageal continuity even when a high degree of tension of the anastomosis was present, due to unfavorable anatomic conditions (distance between esophageal pouches greater than or equal to three dorsal vertebrae). A partial leak was observed in 6.3 % of cases.

In our experience, the use of fibrin sealant has proved to be of great interest. In particular, in esophageal surgery it has two fundamental roles: sealing

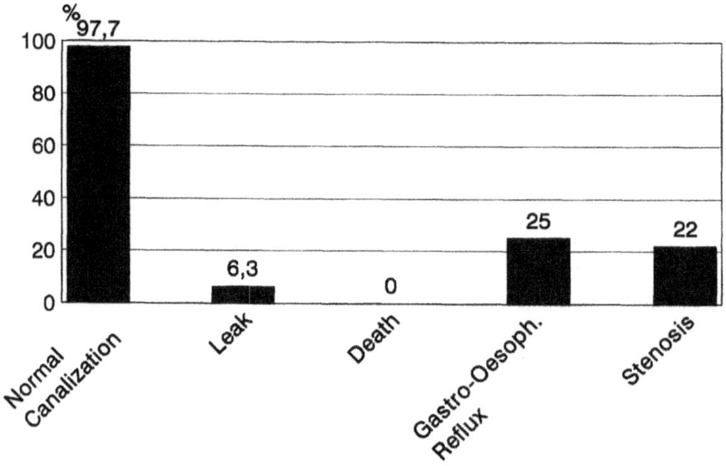

Fig. 1. Results in patients after surgery (*n*–95)

and consolidation. As it acts in a very short time, an immediate effect follows application on sutures or anastomoses [8], and thus it is possible to obtain rapid consolidation and a reduction of the risks of bacterial contamination and leakage. Moreover, fibrin sealant is a homologous plasma derivative and thus does not produce abnormal tissue reactions; it stimulates the normal restoration process and is subsequently resorbed by normal tissue enzyme systems.

References

1. Ahmed A, Spitz L (1986) The outcome of colonic replacement of the esophagus in children. Prog Pediatr Surg 19: 37–54
2. Howard R, Mayers NA (1965) Esophageal atresia: a technique for ologating the upper pouch. Surgery 58: 725–727
3. Lindahl H, Rintala R, Louhimo I (1987) Oesophageal anastomosis without bougienage in isolated atresia – do the segments really grow while waiting? Z Kinderchir 42: 221–223
4. Livaditis A (1973) Esophageal atresia: a method of overbridging large segmental gaps. Z Kinderchir 13: 298–306
5. Mayers NA, Neasly SW, Auldest AW, Kent M, Wright V, Chetcuti P (1981) Oesophageal atresia without fistula-anastomosis or replacement. Pediatr Surg Int 2: 216–222
6. Puri P, Blake N, O'Donnell B, Guiney EJ (1981) Delayed primary anastomosis following spontaneous growth of esophageal segments in esophageal atresia. J Pediatr Surg 16: 180–183
7. Rehbein F, Schwedwe N (1971) Reconstruction of the esophagus without colon transplantation in cases of atresia. J Pediatr Surg 6: 746–752
8. Thorson GK (1983) The role of the tissue adhesive fibrin seal in esophageal anastomosis. J Surg Oncol 6: 112–116
9. Waterston DJ, Bonham Carter RE, Aberdeen E (1962) Oesophageal atresia: tracheo-oesophageal fistula. A study of survival in 218 infants. Lancet 1: 819–822

The Etiopathogenesis of Intra-Abdominal Adhesions and Their Prophylaxis with Highly Concentrated Human Fibrinogen

W. Brands, H. Wirth, and H. Schneider-Brown

Abstract

To prevent recurrent intestinal obstructions, we performed sutureless plication of the small bowel with fibrin adhesive only.

In our 31 patients, aged from 6 h to 13 years, there were four patients who had undergone surgery for laparoschisis, 15 children with recurrent adhesion ileus after intestinal resection or appendectomy, three patients with primary peritonitis, six children who had undergone surgery for necrotizing enterocolitis, and three patients with perforation in intestinal atresia. Excluded were those patients who had local and limited adhesions or serosa defects in which sealing with fibrin adhesive was also performed.

In all patients minimal and dense adhesions were totally lysed. Then the small bowel was joined together in loop lines, and the plication was fixed by fibrin adhesive. The remaining lesions of the serosa were also sealed with fibrin glue (Tissucol). In comparison to patients with mesenteric plication of Childs and Phillips ($n = 14$), patients treated with fibrin adhesive plication did very well, and the postoperative course was uncomplicated, especially with no further evidence of obstruction.

Clinical experience suggests that highly concentrated human fibrinogen is able to induce healing of serosa lesions and to prevent intra-abdominal adhesions from developing. Furthermore, it must be stressed that the procedure is time saving and easy to perform. Above all, the high risk of tissue necrosis or intestinal perforation due to ischemia by sutures and stitches observed with the traditional technique of plication can be avoided.

Introduction

Recurrent intestinal obstruction due to adhesions has become an increasingly common problem as the number of operations and reoperations grows. The formation of undesirable adhesions after laparotomies remains an unsolved problem. About 3 % of all surgery patients have to be subsequently relaparotomied due to adhesions ileus.

In 1937 Noble [7] introduced the serosa to serosa plication and in 1960 Childs and Phillips [3] introduced the transmesenteric "knitting needle" plication. Both procedures create "planned" adhesions in an attempt to prevent future obstruction episodes. The use of inner intestinal splints with long tubes is a further possibility in prophylaxis of adhesion ileus [10], as is the intra-abdominal application of various substances [5, 9]. All these methods, however, are associated with some degree of complications.

In our earlier investigations of the disintegration of inserted fibrin and the protective effect against lysosomal enzymes released from tissue necrosis, we performed small-bowel plication with fibrin adhesive in cases of recurrent intestinal obstruction only in the region of detached adhesions. Local serosa defects are likewise sealed with the glue [1, 2]. Experiments in rats confirm the prophylactic effect and support the claims for fibrin adhesive in peritoneal adhesions.

Material and Method

In the prevention of adhesions and adhesive intestinal obstruction after abdominal surgery we have performed sutureless plications of the small bowel with fibrin adhesive over the past 13 years.

A total of 31 patients aged from 6 h to 13 years were treated with a total fibrin plication of the small intestine after adhesion ileus. They all had severe serosa lesions after adhesiolysis or serosa lesions with additional adhesion-promoting factors (peritonitis, among others). Compared with 14 children [10] treated with the conventional technique of mesenteric-plication after Childs and Phillips, there were no procedure-related complications whatsoever in the children in whom fibrin plication was performed. Two children died, their deaths not being related to surgery, but to the sequelae of severe concomitant diseases.The remaining patients were completely free of symptoms directly after surgery and during the further course.

In all patients in the clinical study minimal and dense adhesions were totally lysed. Thereafter the small bowel was joined together in loop lines, and the plication was fixed by fibrin adhesive (Fig. 1). The still released lesions of the serosa were also sealed with the fibrin glue. After the procedure the plication was reposed in the abdomen and, in particular, no subileus or adhesion symptoms were observed. Postoperative X-ray controls revealed a free, undelayed gastrointestinal passage (Figs.2, 3). In one patient with total plication of the small intestine, a later relaparotomy unrelated to ileus revealed no adhesions and, specifically, no more plication.

Discussion

Since exogenously administered fibrin is completely broken down in the abdominal cavity, the clinical application of human fibrinogen for adhesion prophylaxis is possible in the procedures mentioned above.

On the whole the development and spread of adhesions are the result of a multifactorial process (Fig. 4). A key to this process is the shift of the physio-

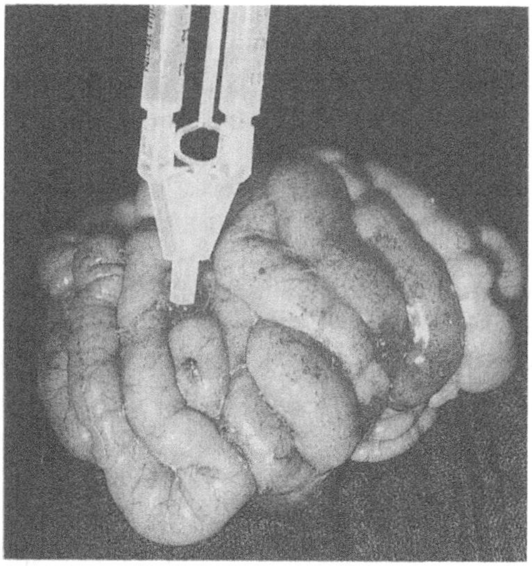

Fig. 1. Fibrin plication in an infant

logical equilibrium between fibrinogenesis and fibrinolysis in favor of fibrinogenesis, the secondarily formed fibrin net being the decisive guide for the invasion and proliferation of fibroblasts.

A mechanical or hypoxemic lesion of the serosa is already caused by surgical trauma, so that an inflammatory reaction subsequently occurs with all its sequelae, i.e., adhesions. The serosa cover cells of the peritoneum, i.e., mesothelium, do not represent a rigid tissue group but are subject to consider-

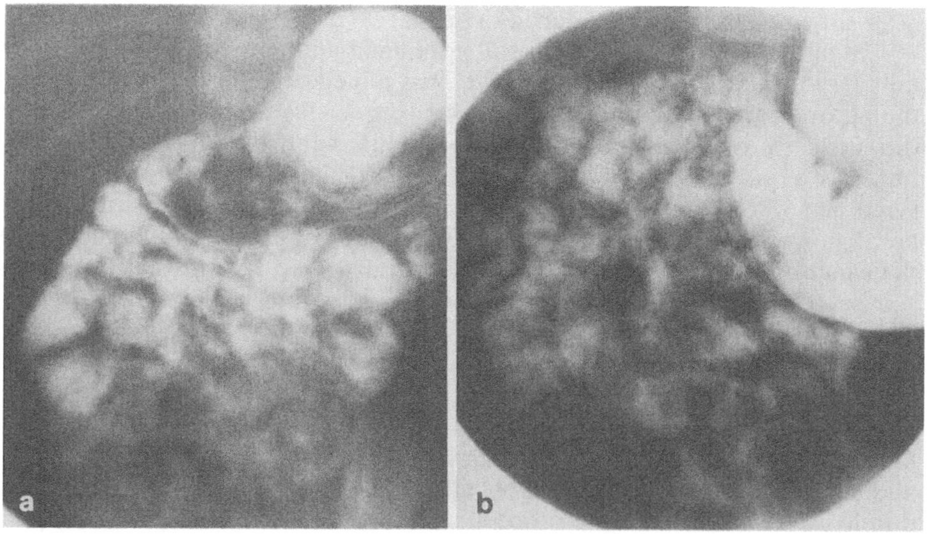

Fig. 2a, b. Postoperative gastrointestinal X-ray control after fibrin plication in an infant. After 1 week (**a**) an 3 weeks (**b**)

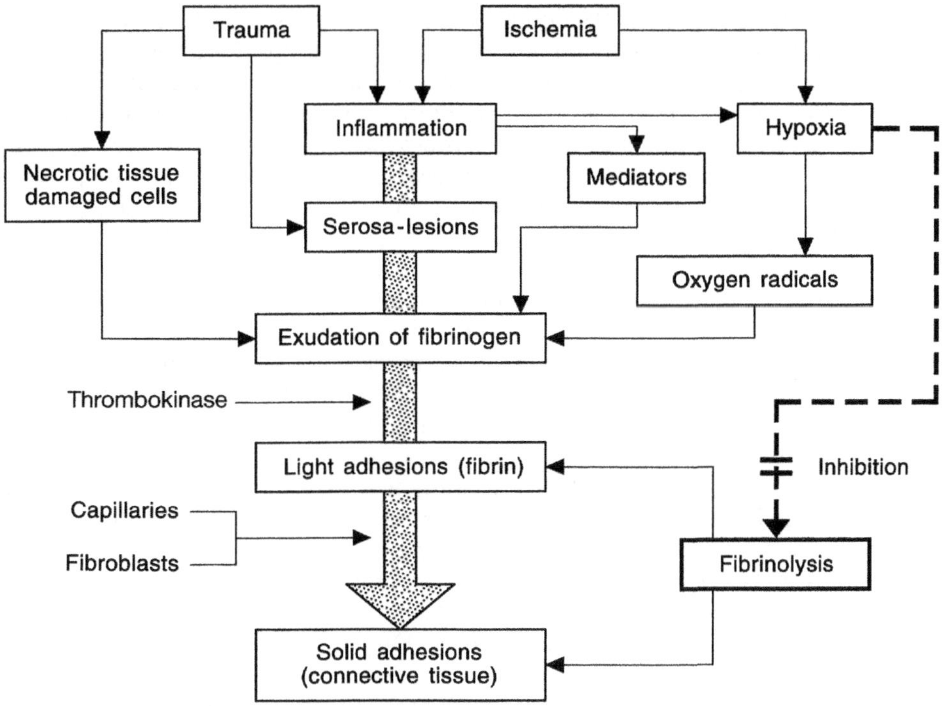

Fig. 3. Simplified overview of the pathogenesis of adhesions

able inflammatory transformation. The cover cells can contract and spread again, thus being able to transform into fibrocytes in response to inflammatory stimuli. Although it is known that two epithelial layers cannot normally adhere to each other, the mesothelium is the exception to this rule. For example, if two intestinal loops are fixed, the dividing serosa coat disappears, resulting in their permanent fixation. Furthermore, one must assume that the so-called milky spots found deep inside the peritoneum, in which primary cells of the immune system as well as a multitude of undifferentiated mesenchymal cells and fibroblasts occur, can, when appropriately stimulated, migrate from the milky spots to the surface and therefore become partly responsible for the connective tissue reconstruction of the fibrin net. The transformation of the mesothelial cells into collagen fibers particularly occurs when these cells are torn from their tissue group, as occurs in the case of detachment of adhesions or traumatic manipulation on the intestinal surface. In the event of even the most minor traumatic lesions to the peritoneum, all of the reactions of nonspecific inflammation can ensue, e.g. vasodilation with increased permeability, migration of granulocytes and monocytes, as well as simultaneous activation of the complement kinin system, among others. The contraction of the vascular endothelium and the associated increase in permeability to cells or fibrinogen depends on the activity of released enzymes. This process can be observed in mechanical trauma or in cell necrosis with destruction of the cell membrane, various enzymes being released. The so-called inflammation mediators play a not inconsiderable role – fibrin fission products having among other things a leukotactic action, thus potentiating the inflammatory reactions, such as increased exudation of fibrin, which in turn activates the coagulation cascade. The complement system also involved consists of several proteins which, similarly to the coagulation after initial activation, trigger a cascade of individual reactions, these reactions preferably taking place on the surface of infiltrated pathogens or body cells. The destruction of endogenous tissue, e.g., endothelial cells, is linked to complement activation. This destruction releases lysosomal enzymes from the cell fragments, especially from granulocytes. Transferred to peritonitis and ileus, this brings to mind the general inflammatory reaction, where inductors of the inflammatory chain are detectable, among others, C 3, C 5, and anaphylatoxin. Overall, after activation of all factors, the complement causes osmotic cell lysis, which means that fission products of the cells can already exert a chemotactic action on leukocytes, resulting in an increase in phagocytosis and degranulation as well as exocytosis of lysosomal enzymes. The lysosomal system mainly serves intracellular digestion. If these enzymes are released, the cell dies. The normal trauma of surgery such as manipulation of the intestines itself already leads to a rise in elastase, which can serve as a marker for the release of lysosomal enzymes, this elevation being up to three times normal levels. Under normal conditions, these released enzymes are neutralized by reactions with their inhibitors, e.g., antithrombin III. These inhibitors are inactivated by complex binding with lysosomal enzyme and by oxidative denaturation by means of oxygen radicals. This fact suggests that nonphysiological amounts of lysosomal enzymes are released when adhesions are surgically removed, so that the capacity of the inhibitors is no longer sufficient, enabling new adhesions to develop after adhesiolysis. This effect is further promoted by ischemia and the inflammatory changes which commonly occur from surgery of adhesion ileus. As soon as 1 h after cell death, tissue-damaging lysosomal enzymes are known to be released and even destroy collagen fibers. Since lysosomal enzymes can cleave antithrombin III, the most important inhibitor of the coagulation system is missing, i.e., fibrinolytic activity is too low, thus facilitating the transformation of the superficial fibrin net into an adhesion loaded with connective tissue.

One decisive factor in the development of adhesions is the presence of oxygen radicals, i.e., the disequilibrium between proteinases and their inhibitors is further increased by the fact that activated phagocytes can produce relatively large amounts of reactive oxidants. In order to be able to produce these oxidants, the phagocytes are equipped with a specific enzyme system, reduced nicotinamide-adenine dinucleotide phosphate (NADPH) oxidase/myeloperoxidase. This NADPH oxidase is a membrane-associated enzyme complex which in combination with an explosive activation of the respiratory chain, the so-called respiratory burst, is responsible for the production of O_2 and H_2O_2. Specifically for the lysosomal enzymes, the oxygen radicals cause an inactivation of the inhibitors of these enzymes and thus lead to their potentiation and a prolongation of their action.

Ultimately, all of the factors mentioned in the development of adhesions are subject to the term amplification, i.e., a key event sets a multitude of reactions in motion which further potentiate each other by feedback and can accelerate the course of the entire inflammatory complex. The first ignition is additionally triggered by a very high degree of granulocyte and macrophage degranulation, so that the concentration of inhibitors is probably then exceeded, the proteolytic activity of the released enzymes destroying tissue and thus additionally activating other systems. In order to prevent the development of adhesions or to break this vicious circle of disturbed equilibrium between proteinases and inhibitors, "causal" adhesion prophylaxis is only possible if the serosa is not damaged or, immediately after damage to the serosa, these chain reactions are halted. This is the case if directly after damaging the serosa, for example, after surgical adhesiolysis, exogenous fibrin is applied to the serosal defects in the hope of getting a headstart on the local, i.e., endogenous, fibrin production, thus eliminating all tissue-damaging (adhesion-promoting) reactions.

Fibrin glue on the damaged serosa thus inhibits fibrin exudation and the reactive course of multiple inflammatory mechanisms, keeping the adjacent surfaces at a distance. Moreover, the release of lysosomal enzymes is braked and the activation of the complement system prevented. Additionally, the activation of free fibroblasts can be precluded, so that random formation of new connective tissue is prevented. Finally, no major inflammatory edema occurs, thus preventing any associated tissue hypoxia. The access of mediators to the target organs is also inhibited so that, as a result of the sealant function of human fibrinogen the pathogenetic course (edema → hypoxia → oxygen-radicals → tissue-damage → triggering of nonspecific inflammatory reactions) is not set in motion and the development of adhesions is ultimately prevented.

Conclusion

To prevent recurrent intestinal obstruction we performed a sutureless plication of the small bowel with fibrin adhesive only. It is also possible to seal detached adhesions with fibrin glue by laparoscopy in prevention of future recurrent adhesions. Clinical [2] and experimental data [4, 6, 8] suggest that highly concentrated human fibrinogen is able to start the healing of lesions of the serosa to prevent adhesions prospectively. Here there is not the high risk of tissue necrosis and intestinal perforations due to ischemia by sutures and stitches as there is in the conventional technique of plication. Furthermore it must be mentioned that the procedure is time saving and easy.

Particularly for use in infants the nontraumatizing procedure is to be stressed and presents a "physiological" principle in the repair of serosa lesions.

References

1. Brands W, Joppich I, Lochbühler H (1982) Anwendung von hochkonzentriertem Human-Fibrinogen in der Kinderchirurgie – ein neues Therapieprinzip. Z Kinderchir. 35: 159
2. Brands W, Diehm T, Lochbühler H, König M, Stock M (1990) Die Anwendung des Fibrinklebers zur Prophylaxe und Therapie intraabdomineller Adhäsionen. Chirurg 61: 22–26
3. Childs WA, Phillips RB (1960) Experience with intestinal plication and proposed modification. Ann Surg 152: 258
4. Larsson B, Fianu S, Jonasson A, Rodriguez-Martinez H, Hedström CG, Thorgirsson T (1986) The use of Tisseel (Tissucol) – a two-component fibrin-sealant in operations for fertility as a sealant and for prevention of adhesions: an experimental study and a preliminary clinical evaluation. In: Schlag G, Redl H (eds) Gynaecology and obstetrics-urology. Springer, Berlin Heidelberg New York, p 90 (Fibrin sealant in operative medicine, vol 3)
5. Minju L, Erchang T (1983) Tierexperimentelle Untersuchungen zur Prophylaxe von Adhäsionen und Adhäsionsileus nach intra-abdominalen Operationen. Acta Acad Med Wuhan 3: 77
6. Lindenberg S, Lauritsen JG (1984) Prevention of peritoneal adhesion formation by fibrin sealant. An experimental study in rats. Ann Chir Gynecol 73: 11
7. Noble TB (1937) Plication of small intestine as prophylaxis against adhesion. Am J Surg 35: 41
8. Oka H, Harrison RC, Burhenne HJ (1982) Effect of a biologic glue on the leakage rate of experimental rectal anastomoses. Am J Surg 143: 561
9. Treutner KH, Winkeltau G, Lerch MM, Stadel R, Schumpelick V (1988) Prophylaxe postoperativer, intraabdomineller Adhäsionen: Substanzprüfung mit einem neuen, standardisierten und objektivierten, tierexperimentellen Modell. In: Schriefers KH, Messmer K, Schwaiger M (eds) Chirurgisches Forum 1988 für experimentelle und klinische Forschung, vol 105. Springer, Berlin Heidelberg New York, p 463
10. Waag KL, Menardi G, Brands W (1980) Mesenterialplikatur und innere Dünndarmschienung bei rezidivierenden postoperativen Adhäsionen im Kindesalter. Z Kinderchir 30: 46

Fibrin Sealing in Circumcision

W. A. MAIER

Abstract

There are a large number of uses for fibrin tissue glue in pediatric surgery. Besides its many applications in gastrointestinal, thoracic and reconstructive surgery we have also used fibrin tissue glue for simple pediatric surgical procedures that are routinely performed at the Clinic of Pediatric Surgery at Karlsruhe.

In children, circumcision of the foreskin is performed by means of a Gomco clamp. While in the past the cut area lying between the long circumference of the glans and the sulcus coronarius was closed with interrupted sutures, the method of choice is now fixation with fibrin tissue sealant, which guarantees smooth borders and a highly satisfactory cosmetic result. This method has been being used for approximately 10 years and the results have been excellent.

Introduction

Circumcision of the prepuce is in itself not a subject of scientific interest, but perhaps it deserves certain attention with regards to the practicability of using fibrin sealing (Figs. 1, 2).

As circumcision in newborns, infants, and young boys is a daily routine, there is no need to explain the operative techniques. However, a few words might be necessary to explain the contribution of fibrin sealing in this minor operation.

How one should proceed with the circumcision and how much prepuce can or must be removed are questions of individual ideological, religious, and personal opinion.

Materials and Methods

As far as the technique of circumcision is concerned, there are rather different methods. This minor operation is done under general, sacral or local anesthesia.

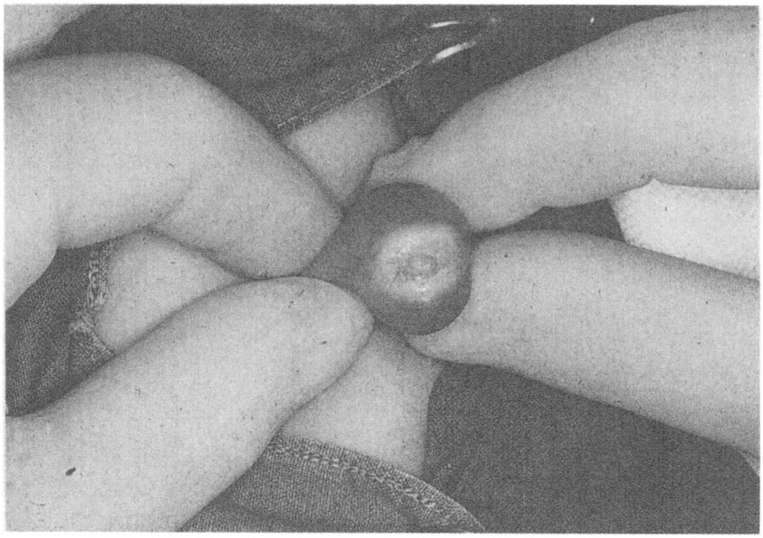

Fig. 1. High degree of secondary phimosis with constricted opening of the prepuce

The classical oblique, oval circumcision with the scalpel has now been replaced by, for instance, the so-called Plastibel method (Richter; Bremen, Germany) or with circumcision after clamping both layers of prepuce with a Gomco clamp, which we use.

The latter method of clamping the two layers of the prepuce using a Gomco clamp (Richter; Bremen, Germany) is an adequate and very easy one:

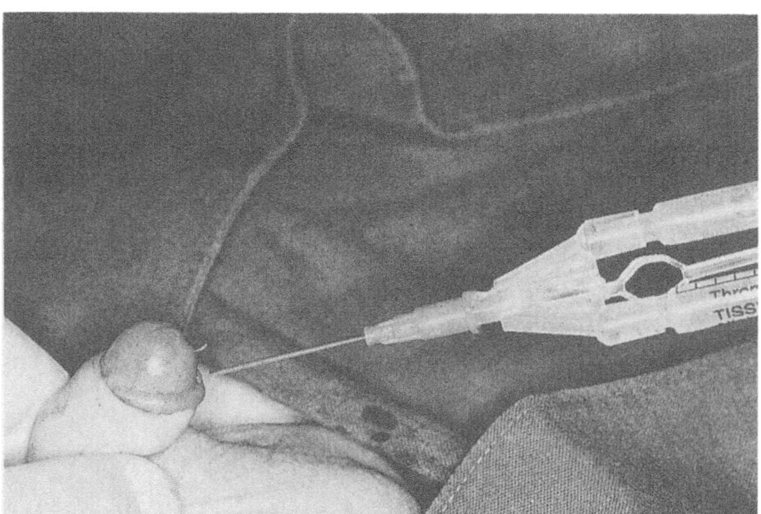

Fig. 2. The application of the two components of Tissucol (fibrin sealant)

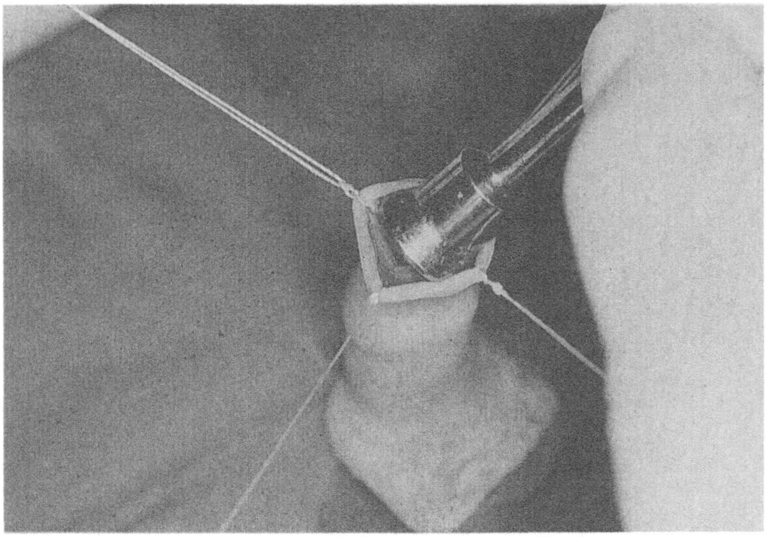

Fig. 3. Placing the piston of a Gomco clamp into the prepuce sack

after a period of 10 min during which the penile skin is clamped, it is possible to immediately perform the circumcision (Figs. 3–5).

Sometimes, unfortunately, the contused layers of prepuce separate from one another immediately or in the first few postoperative hours. Then bleeding occurs, which is unpleasant and can also be very frightening for parents, especially if it happens at night.

Therefore, to avoid this complication when using a Gomco clamp procedure, it is recommended that the newly formed prepuce edge be fixed with fine, interrupted stitches or with a continuous suture.

In the Pediatric Surgical Clinic in Karlsruhe, Germany, over the last 12 years the procedure with stitches has been abandoned and instead the newly formed edge has been sealed with fibrin tissue glue, a method in which the wound area dries very fast and, most importantly, it ensures smooth cut edges, leaving a cosmetically acceptable, adequate result (Figs. 6, 7).

Results

It can not be denied that the cosmetic aspect must also be taken into account in circumcision. Fibrin tissue glue (we always use Tissucol[1]; Immuno, Vienna) dries within 2–3 min and no further steps are required (Figs. 8, 9).

Finally, a bandage, for instance, a Fixomull (Beiersdorf; Hamburg, FRG) stretch bandage or similar product, should be adapted and the small penis should be put in an erect position for 24 h at least. This gives additional protec-

1 Tissucol Duo S, human fibrinogen, human thrombin, steam treated

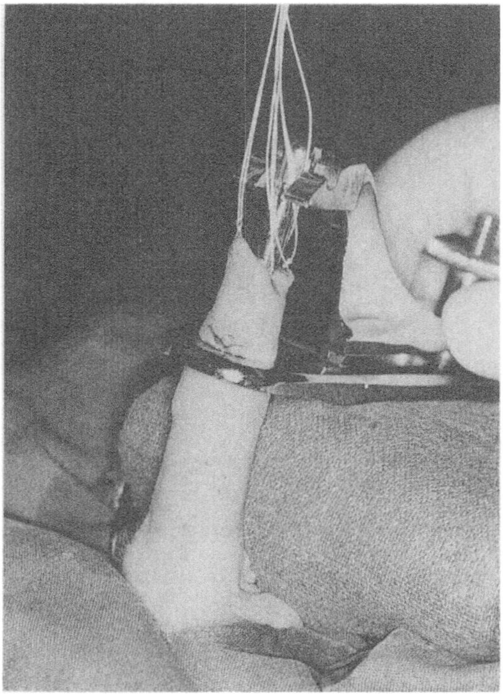

Fig. 4. The piston is now screwed together with the baseplate of the Gomco clamp: begin of the clamping

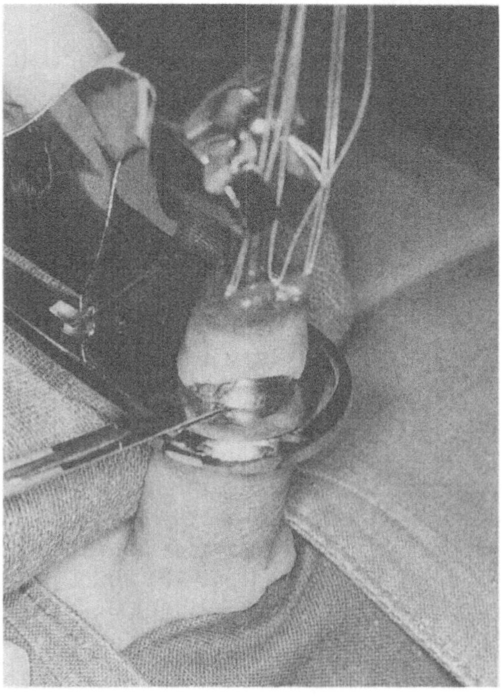

Fig. 5. Resection along the piston

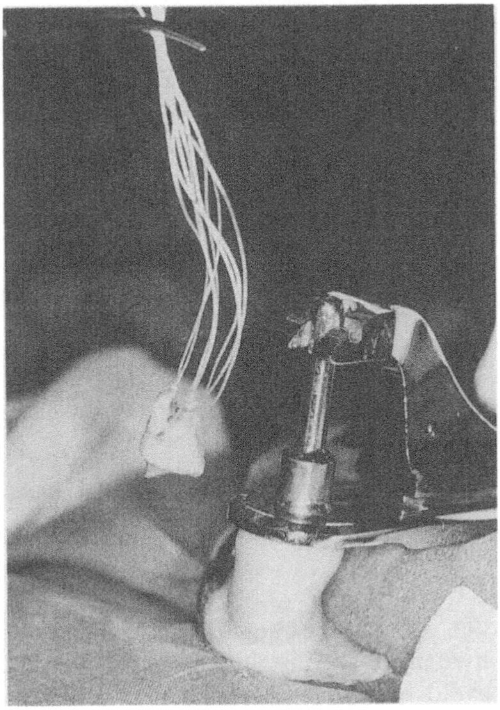

Fig. 6. Resection is complete

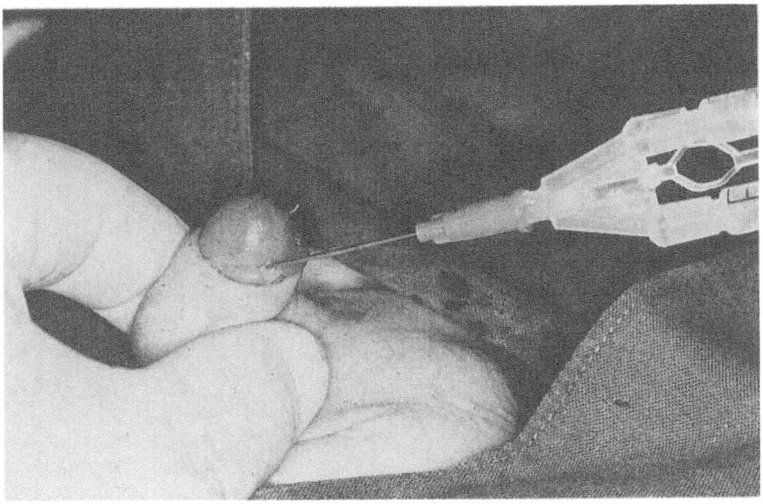

Fig. 7. The application of Tissucol (fibrin sealant) stops any bleeding and seals the edge of both prepuce layers

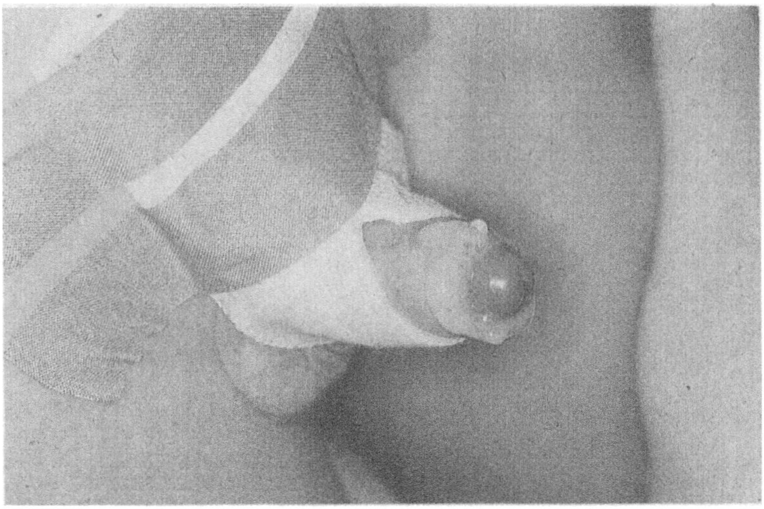

Fig. 8. The postoperative bandage and position of the penis

tion to the circumcised prepuce in the immediate postoperative period and thereafter. During the postoperative phase of the first 3 days, it is necessary to avoid contact with underwear and, wherever possible, with diapers. Little boys, 2–8 years old, should not be allowed to walk around very much in the first 2–3 days.

On the fourth or fifth day, the circumcised child may have a bath. If a little camomile extract is added to the bathwater, this ensures fast and uncomplicated wound healing (Fig. 10).

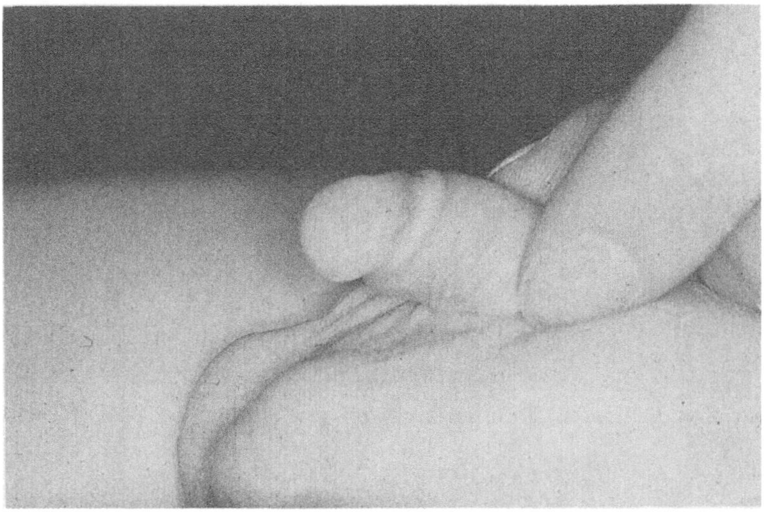

Fig. 9. An early result 2 weeks after complete circumcision

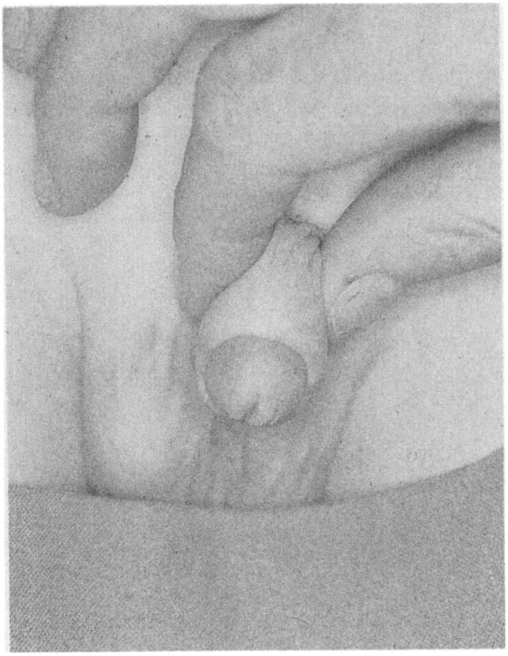

Fig. 10. Largest circumference of the glans

The figures should have adequately demonstrated the method of applying fibrin sealant and the very good results achieved. Undoubtedly, especially in countries where circumcision is done on religious grounds, countries which are often quite poor, the methods described here may not be necessary, as post-operative bleeding is not considered as serious. However in the countries of the Western world, this plays an important role, and in addition to the efforts made to minimize bleeding, efforts are also made to make the cosmetic outcome as positive as possible.

Conclusion

Since it was first reported, fibrin sealing in circumcision has found widespread acceptance and, importantly, can be used very economically. The cosmetic outcome, too, means that the further spread of this method is desirable.

Subject Index

Springer-Verlag and the Environment

We at Springer-Verlag firmly believe that an international science publisher has a special obligation to the environment, and our corporate policies consistently reflect this conviction.

We also expect our business partners – paper mills, printers, packaging manufacturers, etc. – to commit themselves to using environmentally friendly materials and production processes.

The paper in this book is made from low- or no-chlorine pulp and is acid free, in conformance with international standards for paper permanency.

GPSR Compliance

The European Union's (EU) General Product Safety Regulation (GPSR) is a set of rules that requires consumer products to be safe and our obligations to ensure this.

If you have any concerns about our products, you can contact us on ProductSafety@springernature.com

In case Publisher is established outside the EU, the EU authorized representative is:

Springer Nature Customer Service Center GmbH
Europaplatz 3
69115 Heidelberg, Germany

Batch number: 10704771

Printed by Printforce, the Netherlands